The
PRESCRIBED DRUG GUIDE
A Holistic Perspective

DEDICATION

To my wife, Hilary, for all her love and support

STEPHEN GASCOIGNE
M.B., Ch.B., C.Ac., Dip.C.H.M.

The
PRESCRIBED DRUG GUIDE
A Holistic Perspective

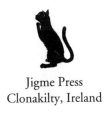

Jigme Press
Clonakilty, Ireland

Published in Ireland by

JIGME PRESS

Glebe House, Ardfield, Clonakilty, Co. Cork, Ireland
Email: *info@drgascoigne.com*
Website: *www.drgascoigne.com*

© Stephen Gascoigne, 2003

ISBN 0 9522189 4 1

British Library Cataloguing in Publication Data
A catalogue record for this book is available from the British Library.

This book contains general information only. It does not contain personal health advice. The content of this book is never a substitute for the advice of a competent medical practitioner. In particular, it may be dangerous to stop taking medication without first obtaining professional advice. The author accepts no liability for injury, loss or damage to anyone acting on foot of the content of this book. Any person who does so, does so entirely at his or her own risk. No responsibility is accepted for any errors or omissions in the contents of this book.

Printed by Antony Rowe, Chippenham, UK
Cover design and typesetting by Declan O'Donovan
Cat logo by Rob Hopkins
Proofreading and indexing by Gloria Greenwood

Contents

Contents

ACKNOWLEDGEMENTS

I owe my thanks to many people during the process of writing this book
but especially to:

Hilary Gascoigne, Gloria Greenwood, Rob Hopkins for his artwork,
Carey Horvath, Carol Schofield, Declan O'Donovan

HOW TO USE THE BOOK

This book provides clear and accessible information about prescribed drugs. It is primarily aimed at practitioners of holistic medicine but I would hope that patients, themselves, could be fully informed of the uses, misuses and effects of drugs. In this way, people can decide upon treatment that is appropriate for them in full knowledge of the possible effects. This text is a companion to *The Clinical Medicine Guide – A Holistic Perspective*,[1] which describes diseases, their symptoms, treatment and holistic management in some detail.

The first four chapters of *The Prescribed Drug Guide* lay down the basis for dealing appropriately with patients who take prescribed drugs. In addition, I classify drugs according to their strength of action. This is a method of determining which drugs must never be reduced or withdrawn and which drugs can be reduced in selected cases.

The remainder of the book presents information about prescribed drugs[2] themselves. In this book, I focus on drugs that are commonly used in outpatient practice. I do not include information about injectable drugs. The drugs are classified according to the diseases treated (e.g. Chapter 7 deals with drugs that treat asthma). Drug information is listed according to the following:

- Generic name[3]
- Brand (trade) name[4] – There may be several different brand names for each generic named drug according to the pharmaceutical company that markets each brand. Brand names may differ from country to country and I have included those used in the UK, Ireland, the USA, Australasia and South Africa. The list of brand names is comprehensive and exhaustive but there may be some missing due to changes since publication. Please consult *www.drgascoigne.com* for the latest information. Any brand name that is followed by an asterisk (*) contains more ingredients than the generic drug name mentioned there. For example, 'Distalgesic' is listed on pages 172 and 175 because it contains paracetamol and an opiate.
- Dosage – This refers to the usual dosage given. Confusion can arise when trying to compare dosages of different drugs. For example, some people think that 5 mg of Valium (see page 195) is less strong than 10 mg of temazepam. However, this is not comparing like with like, just as a pint of whiskey cannot be compared with half a pint of beer. The dosages quoted are for adults, unless otherwise stated.

- Uses
- When not to be used
- Cautions
- Effects – These are grouped into different systems to make them easier to read. I have grouped drugs together, as related drugs have similar effects. For example, on page 197, the effects of benzodiazepines are listed as a group, rather than covering each one individually.[5] I have translated most medical terms into everyday language to make them easy to follow, but a medical dictionary may also be useful.

Some general comments can be applied to all drugs regarding the following areas.

When not to be used – No drug should be given to anyone who has an allergy or sensitivity to that drug or ingredients mixed with it.

Cautions – Many drugs are hazardous in pregnancy and while breast-feeding. In my opinion, no drug should be taken at these times unless it is a life-threatening situation.

Effects – Any drug that causes drowsiness, tiredness, fatigue, dizziness, loss of balance, sedation and so forth may interfere with the person's ability to operate machinery or to drive. Anyone taking such a drug must not operate machinery or drive until their reaction to the medication is known.

I include comments from a holistic perspective based upon my experience of treating patients with Chinese medicine for the last 20 years, so that practitioners can have some guidance about how to deal with such medications. I have included cases from my own practice to show how drug withdrawal can proceed, when judged appropriate. These cases also include details of treatment by means of Chinese medicine. I hope this does not deter practitioners of other modalities from using this information. The point I am making is that it is possible to manage patients who are taking prescribed drugs and for them to reduce their medication when receiving holistic treatment.

There are comprehensive indexes at the back of the book so that you can find information easily and quickly. All the information in this book is supported by my website (*www.drgascoigne.com*), which also offers supervision, support and services to practitioners of holistic medicine. A final chapter discusses the energetic qualities of prescribed drugs and may be of interest to practitioners of Chinese medicine.

Notes

1 *The Clinical Medicine Guide – A Holistic Perspective* by Dr Stephen Gascoigne (Jigme Press, 2001).

2 All the information about drugs contained in this book is in the public domain. It is gathered from medical journals, conference reports and presentations, clinical reports and the personal experiences of clinicians. No source of information should be considered to be the final word, as effects of drugs that have not been previously noted are continually being reported.

3 The generic name is the official medical name for the drug.

4 The pharmaceutical company that markets a particular drug gives the brand name. Other companies may market the same, generically named, drug under different trade names, depending on regulations concerning patents and licences. Simply stated, if you can pronounce a drug name it is probably the trade name. For example, Valium is a brand name and diazepam is its generic name. The brand name is often a registered name. All brand names in this book, therefore, are assumed to be registered names and entitled to carry the symbol ® after the name.

5 Many drugs are examples of so-called, 'me-too' drugs. Rival manufacturers produce these after the first patent of a new generic drug. Examples of these include the betablockers – see page 110. Their names all end in '-olol', indicating their relationships. This enables different manufacturers to have their own betablocker for the duration of the patent.

1 INTRODUCTION

A man in his mid-60s is admitted to hospital for observation. He is taking a number of prescribed drugs, including digoxin, a diuretic and tranquillisers. His medication is stopped on admission and he sleeps for most of the next two days. When he wakes up, he feels rested and well. In fact, he feels better than he has felt for years. He continues to be in hospital for a further two weeks, where all investigations prove to be normal. He goes home in a much better condition.

Do not misunderstand my reasons for relating this story, which happened when I worked in hospital practice. I am not advocating that people should stop their medication suddenly or without guidance, but it does suggest that prescribed drugs may not always be as helpful or as problem-free as we are led to believe. Such experiences guide our clinical practice and teach us that prescribed drugs, although sometimes helpful, are frequently over-used, often leading to uncomfortable symptoms and feelings of ill health. My firm belief is that modern medicine has travelled too far down the cul-de-sac of searching for the 'magic bullet' with which to treat disease. The current research into genetics is merely a repetition of this underlying conventional view that such a holy grail can be discovered.

This book is not anti-drug nor anti-doctor, although it may be perceived as such. Drugs are necessary for some people and in some situations. Certain prescribed drugs prevent people from dying or from developing serious complications of a particular disease. However, these situations are relatively uncommon and most people we see in the clinic do not have a life-threatening disease. It is important for practitioners to know which drugs are used in cases of life-threatening disease and these are discussed in Chapters 3 and 20.

Conventionally, of course, it is the disease that is treated and not the patient. There are over 12 million people in the USA with asthma and they are all treated with a selection of the same two or three drugs. There is no individualisation of the treatment and there is little consideration of holistic methods of treatment. The emphasis in holistic medicine[1] is to treat the person as an individual, to work with people and to support their fundamental healing processes. Many prescribed drugs are considered to be 'anti-' something – antidepressants, antibiotics, antihistamines, anticonvulsants. Symptoms are to be removed and suppressed. Again, there are times when this is necessary to preserve life, but we now live in an age where such drugs are over-used and abused.

Any drug that is used to suppress a certain set of symptoms is likely to produce similar symptoms itself.[2] For example, antibiotics are given to kill bacteria, but they cannot differentiate between those bacteria that cause disease and those that are helpful and so they also adversely affect our whole system, leading to increased susceptibility to infection. The word 'antibiotic' means 'against life' – and not just bacterial life. This leads to the common symptoms of tiredness, poor appetite, loose bowels and so on. Another example is penicillamine (page 49). This is used to treat rheumatoid arthritis and yet its side-effects include similar autoimmune disorders, such as systemic lupus erythematosus and dermatomyositis, as well as rheumatoid arthritis itself.

The use of drugs in our society is very common and seems to be increasing. Modern conventional medicine reflects this trend and many people are given prescribed drugs. In the UK, 1 in 12 women and 1 in 25 men regularly take antidepressants. There were 12 million prescriptions for antidepressants in England alone in 2000, an increase of 50% since 1997. In the US, most adults take at least one medication each week, 12% of women over the age of 65 take at least ten medications and 25% take at least five medications. Almost 60% of general medical service patients in Ireland over 65 years of age take more than 2 medications. There are huge numbers of patients taking regular prescription medication and this has significant consequences, not only for health but also financially.

COST OF PRESCRIPTION DRUGS

Health services all over the world are having great difficulty funding prescribed drug use. As each year goes by, the cost rises as newer (and more expensive) drugs become available. The cost of retail prescription drugs in the US was $42.7 billion in 1991 rising to $157.5 billion in 2001. Antidepressants are currently the biggest seller, with $12.5 billion of sales in 2001 in the US alone. Anti-ulcer drugs came a close second with $10.8 billion of sales, an increase of 14.4% on the previous year. Sales of Lipitor, the cholesterol-lowering drug, rose 46% from 1998 to 1999, while sales of all statins (one class of cholesterol-lowering drugs) rose 20%. The National Health Service (NHS) in the UK spends over £6 billion per year on medications. Almost 15% of the NHS budget is spent on prescribed drugs. In 2001, the pharmaceutical industry in the UK exported drugs to the value of £8.9 million. In addition, much more money is spent on over-the-counter remedies.

A story from my own practice illustrates the costs of medications. I saw a patient who was suffering from a severe attack of sinusitis. She had seen her own doctor and been given a course of antibiotics. These made her ill and she returned to be a given a further course of antibiotics. At the end of the week she felt no better and, on a further visit, was given a third course of antibiotics and a corticosteroid nasal spray. She contacted me a week after with the same symptoms as before, except that she felt more tired, lethargic and unwell. The three visits to her doctor cost €75 and the four prescriptions €254, giving a total of €349 (£220 or $US340).

INFORMATION ABOUT PRESCRIBED DRUGS

It is frequently difficult to obtain clear, accessible information about prescribed drugs. People are often not given full information about a particular drug they have been prescribed. Such information, if available, may be difficult to understand or lacking in detail. Representatives of drug companies are an important source of information for general practitioners about prescribed drugs.[3] It can be difficult to obtain information that is free from industry bias. Approximately 50% of authors who write guidelines for clinical practice have some interaction with the pharmaceutical industry.[4] It is pharmaceutical companies that gather information about drugs[5] when they are tested and, although some effects are listed, there may well be many that are not. The bibliography at the end of this book lists useful sources of information about drugs.

Drugs are tested singly, yet, in real life, people are frequently given several drugs at the same time. My father became ill during the writing of this book and I saw at first hand the number and frequency of medications that people are given. He was taking eight drugs several times a day and his early morning routine was to take five different drugs together before breakfast. I would suggest that no one is in a position to know all the interactions and effects of such a cocktail. The effects of drugs when taken with others are not investigated and, although some drug interactions are known, many are not.

There has been no long-term follow-up of people taking drugs to check whether people who take similar drugs for similar diseases develop related conditions later. People may report adverse reactions to their doctor and these may, or may not, be relayed to the relevant authorities. This lack of information and its inevitable confusion pervades the whole area of prescribed drugs.

There are basic misunderstandings about drugs and their actions within both the medical profession and the pharmaceutical industry. Studies are not conducted in the same way as trials for homoeopathic remedies, where a substance is given to groups of healthy people and the symptoms experienced are recorded in their entirety – mental, emotional and physical. These 'provings' are thoroughly documented and present reliable pictures of the effects of the substances tested. Drugs, on the other hand, are given to people who already have symptoms, for indeterminate periods of time and with less detailed recording of their effects. Clinical trials[6] are performed, but there is no interest in the totality of the symptoms produced by each drug. The focus is on one, usually physical, effect.

New drugs are particularly likely to cause problems that are not picked up during trials. A US study of 548 new drugs that were introduced between 1975 and 1999 showed that 56 were either subsequently withdrawn from the market or had warnings attached about the danger of death or serious injury. Half of these problems occurred within the first seven years of the drug's introduction.[7] This is an important source of ill health, as almost 20 million Americans took one or more of the five drugs that were withdrawn between September 1997 and September 1998.

SIDE-EFFECTS

Prescribed drugs are given and taken in order to reduce symptoms. They do not 'cure',[8] in the sense of the term when it is used by practitioners of holistic medicine. According to the principles of holistic medicine, prescribed drugs suppress the symptoms and often merely replace the original condition with another, drug-induced, condition, which may be more severe than the original. This is the origin of so-called 'side-effects'. It is this process which can cause confusion. Instead of seeing the symptoms clearly, a picture emerges that may be due to the drug or (more likely) due to a combination of the drug and the original condition. The study of side-effects can shed some light on what is happening.

The term 'side-effect' can be misleading. All drugs have a particular group of actions specific to that agent. These actions may manifest differently in individual people, but they cannot be avoided. The constipating action of morphine cannot be separated from its sedating one, and you cannot separate the blood pressure lowering effect of betablockers from their effect on circulation of producing cold hands and feet. All of these actions are a result of the drug being administered. It is purely arbitrary, and dependent upon the needs of the moment, to name one action the desired effect and another the side-effect.

According to official figures, up to 40% of people experience side-effects when taking drugs, although my estimate and that of other clinicians would be higher. Around 8% of all hospital admissions are a result of side-effects, although some studies suggest this figure is higher. The drugs most commonly implicated include antibiotics, insulin, prednisolone, anticoagulants, non-steroidal anti-inflammatory drugs, antidepressants, tranquillisers and cardiovascular drugs (e.g. digoxin, diuretics). One report suggests that deaths from non-steroidal anti-inflammatory drugs are the fifteenth commonest cause of death in the US[9] – an estimated 16,500 people, usually dying from gastrointestinal bleeding and ulcers.

There is a significant number of deaths from prescribed drugs. In Norway, over a two-year period, 18.2% of patient deaths were classified as being directly or indirectly associated with one or more drugs.[10] In the USA, prescribed drug use is the fourth commonest cause of death, with over 100,000 deaths occurring per year.[11] In Australia, around 9,000 people die each year as a result of medical misadventure and 50,000 are ill as a result of medical treatment.[12] Estimates show that 30% of hospital patients experience one or more adverse drug reactions. Around 5% of outpatients may require admission to hospital as a result of adverse drug reactions.[13]

The number of side-effects is dependent on several factors. Side-effects are more likely with:

- higher doses;
- multiple drug use;
- the very young and elderly; and
- women (twice as often as men).

It has also been noted that women are twice as likely as men to die as a result of a drug reaction. This may reflect the use of the oral contraceptive pill, which is widespread and has powerful effects.

An important consideration is the route of administration, since certain routes are associated with lower dosages and a lower incidence of side-effects. The routes commonly used, listed from less to more severe, are:

- topical (on the skin, for example);
- by inhalation;
- enteral (oral/rectal); and
- by injection (intravenous/intramuscular/subcutaneous).

A survey of over 2,000 people over the age of 65 in the US revealed that 6.9 million people in the US are given questionable medication, whilst almost 1 million received one or more medications considered inappropriate. These medications included tranquillisers and antidepressants that leave patients feeling 'dazed, groggy or susceptible to falls'.[14]

Simple errors in prescribing also add to the dangers from side-effects. Such errors are common and can occur in almost 20% of medication doses. They include giving the wrong dose, giving the medication at the wrong time, giving patients other drugs and forgetting to give medication. Almost 1 in 10 of these errors (that is, more than 40 in a typical 300-patient unit) could potentially carry serious medical consequences.[15] In Ireland in 2001, 400 errors in drug administration occurred in one hospital alone (Tallaght hospital). In the UK in 2001, 10,000 recorded medicine errors led to 1,100 deaths.

An additional hazard is that drugs are sometimes prescribed outside of their official uses. Many drugs used in children are unlicensed or are prescribed outside the terms of their product licence (off-label).[16] According to data published in the *British Medical Journal*, 13.2% of GPs' prescriptions for children in Germany are off-label and 22.7% in Holland.[17]

ADDICTION

Prescribed drugs cause varying degrees of addiction, although the term 'dependence' may be used nowadays. The degree of dependence associated with a drug depends mainly upon the precise drug given. For example, psychoactive drugs such as tranquillisers, depressants and 'major' tranquillisers quickly lead to dependence and will cause withdrawal syndromes when they are stopped suddenly. In reality, of course, all drugs produce addiction or dependence (i.e. a desire to continue taking a drug for its effect) and withdrawal symptoms are experienced when the drug is reduced in dose or stopped.

It is inevitable that any substance taken regularly can cause dependence. This is because the body adjusts to the constant presence of the substance in question, whether it is coffee, cigarettes or a prescribed drug. Symptoms frequently appear when the substance is taken less often. Energetically, this is known as a release of suppressed symptoms.[18] These have to be dealt with as part of the treatment.

The appearance of withdrawal symptoms is not inevitable and I have seen people who have taken large doses of a drug for long periods of time and are able to stop it, apparently with little trouble. This is, however, the exception rather than the rule and not to be recommended, because strong symptoms can appear suddenly with rapid dose reduction. The consequences can be serious in the case of some prescribed drugs (see Levels 3, 4 and 5, as described on pages 21-24).

Patients are sometimes told that a particular drug is not addictive. This is common with antidepressant medication, especially since it has been recognised that tranquillisers quickly lead to dependence. Antidepressants also are addictive and people often experience withdrawal symptoms if they are stopped suddenly. Medical doctors frequently do not know themselves about the addictive qualities of a drug.

Patients may also be told that a particular drug is 'mild' in its effects. This may or may not be true. I tell people not to confuse a low dose with a mild effect. Although some drugs may be used in relatively low doses, depending on the situation, their effect is not generally mild. I remember a patient with cancer who was told that she was being given a mild form of chemotherapy. Of course, everything is relative, but I, personally, would not describe any form of chemotherapy as mild.

DRUGS AND THE ENVIRONMENT

A source of concern that is rarely addressed is that all pharmaceutical products end up in the environment and are diluted in water supplies. They are often detectable by analysis, although this is infrequently done, so we are generally unaware of what we are ingesting with our daily drinks. Many of these chemicals persist in the environment and have far-reaching consequences for human health, as well as the environment in general. In Germany, for example, Thomas Ternes has found up to 1 ppb of carbamazepine – an anti-convulsant drug – as well as other pharmaceutical agents in samples he has tested.[19]

In the US, about 80% of cancer patients receive chemotherapy drugs for cancer. These chemicals are toxic and are capable of producing cancer. Drugs such as cisplatin and carboplatin are excreted in the urine, up to 70% on the first day of treatment.[20] The rest stays in the body and is slowly excreted over many years. These chemicals are almost unchanged by current sewage treatment methods and therefore remain in the environment, causing untold damage to ecosystems.

SUMMARY

- Prescribed drugs are commonly used in our modern world.
- They are a major source of expenditure in health-care systems.
- They cause side-effects that can range in severity from ill health to death.
- They cause dependence and may lead to withdrawal symptoms if stopped suddenly.

Notes

[1] The term 'holistic' means whole, the whole person. Holistic medicine can include all gentle, non-toxic treatments which seek to see the person as an individual, in a whole way and to provide the means whereby they can become or remain 'whole'. The word 'healing' means, of course, 'to make whole'. Specific forms of holistic medicine include Chinese medicine and other traditional medical systems, e.g. Ayurvedic, Tibetan, native American and so on, herbalism, homoeopathy, osteopathy (particularly cranial osteopathy), chiropractic, naturopathy, aromatherapy, massage and many others.

[2] A basic truth of energy is defined in Newton's third law of motion: 'For every

action, there is an equal and opposite reaction.'

[3] *BMJ* 2001; 323: 378–381.

[4] *JAMA* 2002; 287: 612–617.

[5] A recent survey of medical schools in the US and their relationships with drug companies undertaking drugs trials revealed that standards set up by the International Committee of Medical Journal Editors (ICMJE) are not adhered to. This raises a huge question mark over the validity of data produced by such tests, as they are open to misinterpretation and manipulation because of commercial interests. *NEJM* 347: 1335–1341.

[6] Clinical trials of drugs are usually conducted over a relatively short period of time (say 4 or 6 weeks). There is often a 'placebo run-in' before the main trial, where people who are more likely to respond to a placebo are excluded. Specific groups of people may also be excluded for other reasons. This means that drugs are tested on a pre-selected group.

[7] *JAMA* 2002; 287: 2215–2220.

[8] In energetic medicine, cure is the movement towards a state of balance in the mental, emotional and physical levels of a person. Suppression is the removal of symptoms with no balancing of these levels, leading to a more disordered state than previously.

[9] *Am J Med* 2000; 109: 122–130.

[10] *Archives Internal Medicine* 2001; 161: 2317–2323.

[11] *J Clin Pharmacol* 2000; 40: 1093–1101.

[12] Ron Law, Executive Director of NNFA in New Zealand and member of the New Zealand Minstry of Health Working Group advising on medical error, wrote in an email to the British Medical Journal (*BMJ*, 2000; 321: 1178) of official Australian government reports showing that preventable medical errors in hospitals are responsible for 11% of all deaths, and that 19% of all deaths are caused by medical errors which could have been avoided by the *proper and correct* use of prescribed drugs. Figures for New Zealand are very similar.

[13] *Rational Drug Bulletin* 2001; 11: 1–4.

[14] *JAMA* 2001; 286: 2823–2829, 2866–2868.

[15] *Archives of Internal Medicine* 2002; 162: 1897–1903.

[16] A survey of child psychiatrists and paediatricians in Australia revealed that 45% had prescribed stimulant drugs to children under the age of 5 years. One-third said that they had given drugs that had not been properly tested on children under 12 years. The stimulant, Ritalin, and similar drugs were the most common drugs prescribed, but 60% of the doctors had prescribed Prozac or one of its relatives. More than one-third had instructed patients to take the drugs contrary to the directions on the label. The antipsychotic drug, risperidone, had been used to *treat* aggression.

[17] *BMJ* 2002; 324: 1311–1314.

[18] As drugs are removed or reduced, the symptoms which have been suppressed over

weeks, months or years are released. This is a curative response but may be uncomfortable in some and possibly life-threatening in others. The emphasis must be on how to reduce or remove safely and appropriately.

[19] Christian Daughton and Thomas Ternes, 'Pharmaceuticals and Personal Care Products in the Environment: Agents of Subtle Change?', *Environmental Health Perspectives* 107(6), December 1999.

[20] *The Lost Language of Plants* by Stephen Harrod Buhner (Chelsea Green Publishing, 2002).

2 HOLISTIC MEDICINE AND PRESCRIBED DRUGS

Many patients attending holistic practitioners take prescribed drugs. In my own practice, 30% of patients regularly take prescribed drugs. This complicates treatment and case management, as drugs alter symptoms. In many cases, they lead to further deterioration in health. Holistic treatment and becoming well are both facilitated by the reduction or removal of these chemicals.

A holistic practitioner has a very different view of prescribed drugs to a conventional practitioner. Holistic medicine sees the person as a whole and its aim is to 'cure', in an energetic sense. However, such drugs not only alter symptoms but they can also cause new symptoms to appear. These changes can cause some confusion.

How can the energetic diagnosis be determined, allowing the appropriate treatment to be given? For example, migraine may be characterised by a headache on the left side of the head, throbbing in nature and with feelings of heat in the head and eyes. It may occur each time there is an emotional upset or in the week before a period. The symptoms change when prescribed drugs are given. They may disappear completely or they may be altered in severity, frequency, nature or time of appearance.

There are several ways to deal with this situation.

- Enquire about the original symptoms before the drugs were commenced. This will give a more accurate picture of the underlying energetic condition of the person.
- Compare the person's symptoms with the effects of the drug, as some or all of the person's symptoms may be due to side-effects. For example, a person taking betablockers commonly develops tiredness, chilly hands and feet, impotence and depressed feelings. Such symptoms are the result of the medication.

The particular type of holistic medicine that we practise may determine the precise response.

The patient's presenting symptoms are a combination of the effects of the drug and the person's underlying energetic condition. In general, it is the person's total symptom picture that we need to treat. Having said that, in homoeopathic practice, it is usually more important to consider the situation before the drugs were prescribed in order to arrive at the appropriate homoeopathic remedy. In Chinese medicine, it is the whole picture that is usually treated, by taking account of the original condition and how medication has changed it. A more difficult situation is where the clinical picture completely changes and the symptoms disappear. Here, if possible, the drugs can be withdrawn gradually until symptoms reappear, a case can be taken and a diagnosis made.

Drugs usually interfere with holistic medical treatment for several reasons. They are given in material doses and have powerful actions. They treat merely one symptom and therefore any underlying energetic imbalance is usually worsened. They can directly interfere with holistic methods of treatment. Homoeopaths know that prescribed drugs are one of the most powerful causes of antidoting a remedy (that is, reversal of its action or movement towards disease). This is a particularly Western problem at the moment. In China and societies where drugs are less commonly used, holistic treatment is more effective, acts more quickly and with less difficulties along the way.

Holistic treatment becomes more effective and the process smoother and less complicated as drug dosage is reduced. Interference by the drug and confusion of the clinical picture lessens. This is a helpful situation, since movement is continuing towards health.

As holistic treatment alters the person's condition, the need for the drugs will change. Consider the example of treating someone who has hypertension. The dosage of the drug has to be changed as their blood pressure becomes more normal. In those patients taking thyroxine for hypothyroidism, holistic treatment frequently improves thyroid function. The dosage of thyroxine may have to be reduced as a consequence.

There is a source of potential conflict when holistic practitioners treat people who are taking prescribed drugs. There is a risk that the patient will fall between two contrasting medical systems and become confused by apparently conflicting advice. It is important to avoid the patient becoming a battleground between the philosophies of holistic and conventional medicine. When someone taking prescribed drugs approaches a holistic practitioner, there is clearly a willingness to seek other methods to deal with ill health and uncomfortable symptoms. A large part of holistic treatment is education and providing information – both about the treatment and also about prescribed drugs. When patients are made aware of the options available, they will be in a much better position to decide what they want. The main concern is what is going to benefit the patient.

The responsibility for taking a drug lies with the patient. The patient should never stop or reduce medication on a holistic practitioner's instructions. This could open the way for possible legal repercussions. The patient is the person who must decide, with the benefit of information and support offered by the practitioner.

It is generally respectful and beneficial for a holistic practitioner to communicate about any intended treatment with the prescribing doctor. This is easier if the practitioner already has contact with the doctor and they have a good working relationship. There may be situations where this is not the case or where the patient may not wish there to be any communication with their doctor. This wish must be respected and it is for the practitioner and the patient to decide how best to continue. In more difficult cases, it is certainly helpful to seek out advice and support from more experienced practitioners and from sympathetic conventionally trained practitioners.

SUMMARY

- A holistic practitioner's main concern is what will benefit the patient.
- Prescribed drugs change symptoms – this may cause confusion when making a diagnosis.
- The practitioner should enquire about the original condition.
- It is important to study the effects of the drug being taken.
- Patients should be given information about the medication they are taking.
- It is helpful to liaise with sympathetic, conventionally trained practitioners.

3 HOW TO CLASSIFY THE STRENGTH OF ACTION OF PRESCRIBED DRUGS

The essential question when faced with a patient who is taking prescribed drugs is: 'What is safe and appropriate?' There is a lot of fear and apprehension around the use of drugs. Is it dangerous for patients to reduce their medication?

This depends on the situation, the person and the prescribed drug in question. I have developed a method of classifying prescribed drugs according to their strength of action. Consequently, some drugs can be reduced with care, some need to be taken continually to maintain life, while others are only taken symptomatically.

Prescribed drugs can be assigned to five levels. These levels are not rigid and a drug may appear at another level because of its dosage, length of treatment, the individual patient and the original condition.

LEVEL 1

These drugs are taken occasionally or intermittently for symptom relief.

Disease/Symptom	Drugs used
Pain	Pain relievers (e.g. aspirin, paracetamol)
Indigestion	Antacids
Constipation	Laxatives, faecal softeners
Diarrhoea	Anti-diarrhoeal drugs (e.g. codeine, loperamide)
Minor infections (e.g. tonsillitis, bronchitis, cystitis, etc.)	Antibiotics
Allergic disease	Antihistamines

Table 3.1: Drugs taken for symptomatic relief

Any drug taken symptomatically is included in Level 1. These tend to be mild in their action and are only taken for a short period of time in response to symptoms. They are stopped when the symptom has subsided. Drugs taken in this way do not confuse the case too much, because they are only taken when a symptom appears. As the symptoms improve, there is no further need to take the medication. Antibiotics are included here because they are usually used for minor, self-limiting illness and their effect is one of symptomatic relief.

Any of the drugs listed in Table 3.1 that are taken regularly would be placed in Level 2.

LEVEL 2

The drugs in Level 2 are taken regularly yet pose little or no threat to life if discontinued.

Disease/Symptom	Drugs used
Anxiety	Tranquillisers
Depression	Antidepressants
Arthritis and other musculoskeletal diseases	Non-steroidal anti-inflammatory drugs, sulphasalazine (sulfasalazine), gold, chloroquine, penicillamine
Asthma	Bronchodilators, anti-allergic drugs
Migraine	Anti-migraine medication
Stomach and duodenal ulcers	Anti-ulcer medication
Parkinson's disease	Benzhexol (trihexyphenidyl), levodopa
Inflammatory bowel disease (ulcerative colitis, Crohn's disease)	Sulphasalazine (sulfasalazine)

Table 3.2: Drugs taken regularly

The diseases listed in Table 3.2 comprise most of the work of a holistic medicine practice. In many cases, the drug can be withdrawn or stopped if the underlying condition is treated successfully.

I am not suggesting that people should withdraw their medication rapidly and without supervision. There can be a lot of discomfort involved, even though serious problems may not occur. It is always advisable to reduce medication slowly, so that any flare-up in symptoms can be monitored, managed and treated.

When a disease mentioned in Table 3.2 is more severe, it is more appropriate to consider the drugs to be in Level 3. For example, severe cases of asthma may be treated with several bronchodilator prescriptions together with corticosteroids. This is clearly a more complex case, the approach needs to be more circumspect and any reduction must be managed and slow.

LEVEL 3

The drugs in Level 3 cannot be stopped suddenly when they have been used long-term. The disease itself may be severe (e.g. some cases of autoimmune disease). Generally, however, the diseases in Table 3.3 are merely suppressed by the drug and symptoms alleviated. The difficulty with drugs in this level is that sudden withdrawal may cause problems. For example, long-term corticosteroid use suppresses adrenal function. The adrenals cannot recover if the drug is withdrawn too quickly and there are severe consequences, such as shock, low blood pressure, overwhelming infection and death has occurred in some cases. Betablockers must always be reduced slowly, whether they are prescribed for migraine, anxiety, angina pectoris or high blood pressure.

It is not the disease that is life-threatening, at least not in the short term. It is the long-term use of these drugs that creates a situation where sudden withdrawal is harmful.

Disease/Symptom	Drugs used
Hypertension	Hypotensive drugs
Autoimmune disease	Corticosteroids, immunosuppressants
Angina pectoris	Nitrates, betablockers, calcium channel blockers
Epilepsy	Anticonvulsants

Table 3.3: Drugs taken regularly that cannot be stopped suddenly

I have included epilepsy here because of the risk of epileptic attacks occurring on reduction of the drug. It is unusual for people to die with this condition, although it can happen. More importantly, the appearance of an epileptic attack has far-reaching social and work-related consequences. In addition, there is frequently a lot of pressure for patients to take their anticonvulsant medication. Around 70% of people with epilepsy would not have an attack if they stopped their medication. The difficulty for practitioners is that they do not know if their patient is one of the 70% or not. For this reason, reduction must always be slow and then only in carefully selected cases.

Sudden withdrawal or rapid reduction of the drugs listed in Table 3.3 may cause serious problems, whatever they are used for. With care, in selected cases, they may be slowly withdrawn as improvement begins.

LEVEL 4

These drugs have powerful effects on the mental and/or emotional levels.

Disease/Symptom	Drugs used
Schizophrenia	'Major' tranquillisers and related drugs
Manic depression	Lithium

Table 3.4: Drugs with powerful psychological effects

The conditions listed in Table 3.4 are characterised by mental symptoms that may include lack of insight. In severe cases, there may be delusional symptoms such as paranoia. The drugs in Table 3.4 suppress these mental symptoms. If the drug dosage is reduced inappropriately, there may be a return of these symptoms. Typically, symptoms reappear with full force some four to six weeks after medication has stopped. The patient is no longer in control if lack of insight is a major feature. In-patient care may be necessary, which is not commonly available for those who wish to follow a path of holistic treatment. Unless there is adequate support and follow-up for the patient, a situation may arise which is unmanageable. In addition, the current treatment of psychological difficulties is overwhelmingly drug-based. Certainly, drug reduction is possible in carefully selected cases. Peter Breggin and David Cohen's excellent book, *Your Drug May Be Your Problem*,[1] is an invaluable guide to anyone seeking to reduce these drugs. Even if drug withdrawal is not an option, treatment can definitely benefit patients and ameliorate any side-effects they may experience.

LEVEL 5

These drugs are essential for life and are not frequently seen in everyday clinical practice. They are used in serious life-threatening diseases where they are necessary to keep the patient alive. The patient will die, or certainly be seriously ill, if these drugs are stopped or their dosage reduced inappropriately. The length of time before problems occur depends upon the disease and the drug.

Disease/Symptom	Drugs used
Serious heart rhythm abnormalities, including ventricular arrhythmias	Amiodarone, bretylium, disopyramide, dofetilide, encainide, flecainide, ibutilide, lidocaine, mexiletine, procainamide, propafenone, quinidine, tocainamide
Hypothyroidism	Thyroxine
Diabetes mellitus	Insulin, hypoglycaemic drugs
Hyperthyroidism	Carbimazole, methimazole, propylthiouracil
Diabetes insipidus	Vasopressin, desmopressin
Insufficiency of the adrenal cortex	Fludrocortisone, cortisol[2]
Organ transplantation	Immune system suppressants such as cyclosporin (ciclosporin)
Thrombosis (clotting)	Anticoagulants such as warfarin
Cancer	Chemotherapy agents, immunosuppressants
Severe life-threatening infections such as septicaemia, meningitis	Antibiotics

Table 3.5: Drugs used in life-threatening disease

Patients taking Level 5 drugs can still be treated and side-effects will be ameliorated. The dosage must be maintained, unless there are specific reasons for change based on monitoring or investigations, usually in conjunction with a medically trained practitioner.

Cancer chemotherapy drugs are included because of the difficulty for patients to choose another method of treatment. I have doubts about the effectiveness of chemotherapy in most people with cancer and it is certainly over-used, even from a conventional point of view.[3] Patients need to be motivated and well informed to choose another course of action.

SUMMARY

- Prescribed drugs can be classified into five levels, according to their strength of action.
- Such classification guides the practitioner on which drugs may be reduced or withdrawn in selected cases and which drugs must not be reduced.

Notes

[1] *Your Drug May Be Your Problem: How and Why to Stop Taking Psychiatric Medications* by Peter R. Breggin and David Cohen (Perseus, 1999). Also, *Beyond Prozac* by Dr Terry Lynch (Marino, 2001) is a helpful resource for those seeking information, support and non-drug options for psychological symptoms.

[2] There are several kinds of corticosteroids. These are discussed in detail on page 51. Those used in Addison's disease, such as fludrocortisone and cortisol, are not used in any other situation and should not be confused with corticosteroids used to treat inflammatory disease (e.g. prednisolone), which are included in Table 3.3.

[3] Dr Ralph Moss is a useful source of information, both through his book, *Questioning Chemotherapy* (Equinox, 1995), and his website at www.cancerdecisions.com.

4 PATIENT MANAGEMENT

It is always helpful if the practitioner discusses prescribed drug use with patients. It is a question of clinical judgement to decide when this happens. Many people attend for holistic treatment because they want to come off their medication or because they need help with uncomfortable side-effects. In these cases, it is easy to offer information about prescribed drugs, so that patients can come to an informed decision about their own health. Any such decision must be made as a result of a partnership between the practitioner and the patient. It is the professional role of the practitioner to guide the patient along the most appropriate path towards health. However, practitioners have to respect the patient's wishes and beliefs. The final decision about prescribed drug use must always lie with the patient.

This is more difficult when a practitioner feels that prescribed drugs are interfering with a patient's health and yet the patient does not feel ready to address this. In such cases, it is important to wait, give attention to the patient's needs and support their search for health. At the same time, it is helpful to give people information about any drugs they are taking. However, it is essential that the practitioner's own agendas and biases should not interfere with the attention that the patient needs. If practitioners push a patient towards an outcome based upon their own idea of what is needed, the patient may become unsettled, any curative action of the treatment will be negated and eventually the patient will cease treatment.

GUIDELINES FOR DEALING WITH PEOPLE WHO TAKE PRESCRIBED DRUGS

Is the disease acute[1] or chronic?[2] This is a key question. In cases of acute disease, the practitioner has to see people more often and monitor them more closely. This is particularly true when treating children, as symptoms can change relatively rapidly. However, it is often possible to directly replace prescribed drugs, such as antibiotics, with holistic treatment. There are exceptions to this and these are discussed in Chapter 13.

When dealing with chronic disease, the symptoms will not change rapidly and will not be too strong. It is frequently possible to reduce medication during treatment of the underlying imbalance, bearing in mind the strength of action of the drug in question (as discussed in Chapter 3). This must be managed appropriately, in order to progress with reducing drug medication. A flare-up that cannot be controlled and is very strong will often make the patient lose faith in holistic treatment and return to increased drug medication.

Frequently, what is suspected to be a flare-up is merely withdrawal symptoms from the drugs as they are reduced in dosage. It can be difficult at times to distinguish between worsening of the disease and symptoms that are due to too rapid drug reduction. If the symptoms are relieved quickly by a subsequent increase in drug dosage, this is confirmation that drug withdrawal was causing the symptoms. For these and other reasons, it is important to reduce drug dosage slowly, so that any withdrawal symptoms are minimised.

Prescribed drugs are used to 'control' symptoms. A reduction in dosage may lead to a recurrence or strengthening of symptoms. Therefore, any reduction must be slow and only follow effective treatment by holistic medicine. Essentially, the aim is to replace the medication by holistic treatment. This takes time and must allow for patients to develop faith that holistic treatment is effective. Ultimately, personal experience of the benefits of holistic treatment[3] is the best way for people to learn that medication is not necessary. In this way, people develop confidence that their condition can improve and that there is an effective alternative to drug treatment. Very few patients will reduce or stop their medication on philosophical grounds. In addition, improvement in the patient's condition is confirmation of correct diagnosis and holistic treatment.

Always ask about the original condition for which the drugs were prescribed This may give an indication of the severity of the condition at that time. It can be difficult to ascertain why patients are taking a particular drug. Patients themselves may not know why they are taking a drug: they may not have been told, they may have forgotten or it may be that they were prescribed several drugs together for different conditions. In some instances, a medical practitioner may prescribe drugs inappropriately.

What is the name of the drug? It is helpful to see the actual bottle or container for the drugs. Seeing the printed name on the container will confirm which precise drug is being taken. There are several names for each prescribed medicine but, essentially, there are two that concern us here. There is the generic name and the brand (or trade) name. In this book, all generic names begin with a lower-case letter (e.g. salbutamol), while brand names take an initial capital letter (e.g. Ventolin).

The generic name is the official medical name for the drug. The pharmaceutical company that markets the particular drug gives the brand name. Other companies may market the same, generically named, drug under different brand names, depending on regulations concerning patents and licences. Simply stated, if you can pronounce a drug name it is probably the brand name. For example, Valium is a brand name and diazepam is its generic name.

How strong are the effects of the drug? Always check out the classification of prescribed drugs, as described in Chapter 3. The stronger a drug, the more serious the patient's condition and the more care you will need to take. It may be inappropriate to reduce or stop some drugs and these are generally those in Level 5.

How long has the patient been taking the drug? The situation is easier to deal with if the drug use has been short-term. Clearly, six weeks is much simpler than 16 years!

What dose of the drug is the patient taking? Consult the reference information about the specific drug in question and compare the dosage quoted there with the dose that the patient is taking. It will then be clear whether this a low, medium or high dosage.

How many drugs is the patient taking? Many patients are given several drugs at the same time and this is particularly true in the elderly. It is much easier to deal with one drug than with several, as there will be interactions between them and each has different effects, making it more difficult to thread a way through them.

When faced with a patient who takes several drugs, I generally address the more powerful ones first (bearing in mind that Level 5 drugs, as listed on page 23, cannot generally be easily adjusted). The less powerful drugs can be used as support whilst the stronger drugs are reduced. The patient's health will recover more quickly once the strongest drugs have been dealt with. This is in line with Hering's Law of Cure.[4]

Which is the most powerful drug? This can be assessed using the classification system in Chapter 3, as well as by looking at the side-effects of the drug. Drugs with more severe effects are the most powerful.

Assess the patient's energy The effects of drug withdrawal are much less marked in less serious conditions with strong energy. The process of treatment will also be much smoother. In life-threatening disease, or conditions with the potential to become life-threatening, the practitioner must be very circumspect. The support and help of others may be needed. This is particularly true when the patient takes drugs in Levels 4 or 5.

How much support does the patient have during treatment? The original situation required the use of drugs to suppress symptoms. Is this now the time for these to be released and transformed? The amount of support a patient has is particularly relevant in the case of psychological disorders. The release of suppressed emotional and mental symptoms requires support from family, friends and professionals, as well as the patient's own personal resources.

How much support can you offer your patients? When people begin to reduce their drug dosage, depending on the individual case and the drug involved, they may need a lot of support. You may only visit a town once a week or fortnight and therefore may not be available in the intervening periods. The patient may feel isolated during what can be a very difficult time if support from the practitioner is limited.

What help and support is there for practitioners? It is important that practitioners develop their own system of self-help, professional support[5] and advice. I would consider as a minimum: regular supervision sessions, adequate rest and relaxation, as well as frequent peer group meetings for mutual support. Treatment for the practitioner may also be necessary. It is helpful to consider the professional support and information offered by pharmacists, who are very aware nowadays about prescribed drugs, their uses, contraindications and effects. They are usually supportive of sensible and safe prescribing and frequently are open to alternatives to drug use.

GENERAL RULES FOR DRUG REDUCTION

The first priority of treatment is to see an improvement in the patient's condition. This will confirm that the practitioner's diagnosis and treatment are both correct. It will also increase the patient's confidence in holistic treatment.

After the initial improvement, the drug dosage can be reduced slowly in appropriate cases. This is useful in all cases to avoid a flare-up of symptoms, but is essential when the drugs in question are corticosteroids or other Level 3 drugs. Essentially, the objective is to replace the drug with holistic treatment. The only situation where drug withdrawal should be rapid or immediate is where the drugs that are given are dangerous when used together or if they are causing life-threatening side-effects. These are not common situations, but they do sometimes arise. In an ideal world, the prescribing doctor would not prescribe in such a way and the pharmacist would not dispense such drugs, but such prescriptions can occasionally slip through the net.

There are various ways of reducing drug dosage (see Table 4.1). It is important to try to keep a smooth dosage over the day. For example, if the drug is taken twice morning and evening, it is better to slowly reduce this to one dose morning and evening rather than stopping the evening dose (or the morning) first.

In the case of drugs taken three or four times each day, begin by making gradual reductions in each dosage, and then stop the middle of the day ones first. In this way, the evening and morning dosages that are taken after a long interval are left until last. I would emphasise that flexibility is required here and changes may be made, depending on the situation, the patient, the drug and the condition.

Drug dosage	Possible regime for reduction
2 doses four times daily	Take 2, 2, 1, 2, then 1, 2, 1, 2 and so on
2 doses three times daily	Take 2, 1, 2, then 1, 1, 2 and so on
2 doses twice daily	Take 2, 1 or 1, 2, then 1, 1 and so on
1 dose four times daily	Take 1, 1, 0, 1, then 0, 1, 0, 1 and so on
1 dose three times daily	Take 1, 0, 1, then 0, 0, 1 or 1, 0, 0 and so on
1 dose twice daily	Take 1, 0 or 0, 1 (the missed dose is determined by the patient's symptoms: e.g. if symptoms are worse early in the morning, then maintain the evening dose)
1 dose once daily	Take half a dose once daily
	Take 1 every second day
	Take 1 daily for two days then miss a day
	Take 1 daily for three days then miss a day

Table 4.1: Possible regimes for drug reduction

Most tablets are scored and divide easily. In the case of capsules, it is possible to separate the two halves, divide the powder or granules and replace this in the capsule. It is not wise for people to take just the powder, because of the taste.

A reduction may also be effected if the prescribing doctor gives the same drug in smaller doses (e.g. two 2 mg tablets instead of one 5 mg tablet).

An important point to remember is what *percentage* reduction is occurring each time. For example, if someone taking 2 mg three times daily reduces to twice daily, this is a 33% reduction. However, if their next reduction is from twice daily to once daily, this is now a 50% reduction. Therefore, it may be more appropriate to reduce more slowly, bearing in mind what percentage of the dosage is being stopped. Drs Breggin and Cohen, in their book *Your Drug May Be Your Problem*,[6] talk about a system of dosage reduction where each reduction is by 10%. So, if a patient is taking 20 mg of a drug, they manage drug reduction by taking 2 mg less each time (2 mg is 10% of 20 mg). This is a useful method. However, it is also important to bear in mind that, as the total drug dosage falls, 2 mg will become more and more significant. For example, a reduction from 4 mg to 2 mg is a 50% reduction. It is for this reason that psychoactive drugs in particular can be very difficult to reduce towards the end of the process and that even relatively minor reductions in drug dosage can be difficult to tolerate. Drug dosage can be reduced more quickly with a mild condition, if the dosage is low and the duration of drug treatment is short.

With multiple prescriptions, it can be problematic deciding which drug can be reduced first. In general, it is simpler to reduce one drug at a time, as it can be confusing when too many changes are made to several drugs at the same time. It is more difficult to analyse what is happening. Some practitioners recommend reducing the weakest drug first, so that the patient gains some confidence in drug reduction. However, I generally recommend that patients reduce the strongest drug first (unless it is a Level 5 drug that cannot be changed). This is because it is the most powerful drug that is having the most effect on the patient. For example, in the case of a person with asthma taking corticosteroids and bronchodilators, it is the corticosteroid prescription that has the strongest and most hazardous effects on the system. As the corticosteroid is reduced, the bronchodilators can be used to alleviate any symptoms that arise. If the bronchodilators are reduced first, they may well have to be restarted to deal with any symptoms that arise as the corticosteroids are removed.

Sometimes a drug is used to treat the side-effects of another drug. For example, if a woman is taking hormone replacement therapy (HRT), she may also have to take medication for high blood pressure, which is a common side-effect of HRT. In this case, although HRT is categorised in Chapter 3 as Level 2 and blood pressure medication as Level 3 (and therefore stronger in its effect), it is the HRT that needs to be reduced first. It is important to take each case on its own merits, assess the situation carefully and construct a plan of action for withdrawal of the drug.

SUMMARY

- It is essential to work in partnership with the patient.
- Any drug reduction must be patient-led.
- Gather information about the drugs being taken, their uses and their effects.
- Drug reduction must only take place in selected cases; more care has to be taken in acute situations and instances of severe disease.

Notes

[1] Acute disease may be defined as a disease of rapid onset and short duration (usually with strong symptoms) that either ends in recovery or death. People who have an acute disease know that they are ill. It is clear-cut and indicates that the person is of relatively strong energy. For an acute manifestation to take place there must be strong energy in the system. This is why children tend to have acute illnesses, since their energy is strong.

[2] Chronic disease can be defined as a disease of slow onset and long duration that ends in gradual deterioration of health. The symptoms are more vague than those of an acute problem. This picture indicates that the person's energy is weaker. There are some instances of very few symptoms despite serious chronic disease: for instance, elderly people with bronchopneumonia may have little in the way of cough or fever. They may only present with breathlessness or perhaps confusion.

[3] This is not to say that holistic treatment is the only way in which patients can reduce their medication. There are many ways in which people gain support and strength, thus gathering the resources to address their medication. Holistic treatment is merely another method that may be of benefit to patients. There can be a danger that, just as patients are frequently disempowered and undermined by the use and abuse of prescribed drugs, they may feel equally helpless unless they undertake holistic treatment. The effectiveness of any medical treatment is determined by the degree to which patients, themselves, are empowered to take control and responsibility for their situation.

[4] Hering's Law of Cure is a basic tenet of homoeopathic philosophy and is also true for any method of energetic medicine that leads to cure. It states that cure is the movement of pathology from inside to outside, from above to down, from most important organs to least important, and that symptoms disappear in reverse order of their appearance.

[5] I offer professional support services to practitioners. Details can be seen on my website: *www.drgascoigne.com.*

[6] *Your Drug May Be Your Problem: How and Why to Stop Taking Psychiatric Medications* by Peter R. Breggin and David Cohen (Perseus, 1999).

5 ANGINA PECTORIS

Angina pectoris is pain in the chest due to lack of blood supply to the heart muscle (ischaemic heart disease). There is an association with atherosclerosis. The conventional approach to this condition is to control the pain with drugs and treat any associated raised cholesterol levels.

Treatment (mildest to strongest)	Strength level
Nitrates • symptomatic use • regular use	1 3
Betablockers	3
Calcium channel blockers	3

Table 5.1: Drug treatment for angina pectoris

NITRATES

These drugs relax blood vessels as the nitrate is converted into nitric acid. As the blood vessels relax and open up, the strain on the heart and circulation is eased and so pain is relieved. Nitrates are also used in the treatment of heart failure. There are several of these drugs available – some are taken symptomatically and others are taken regularly. Sudden withdrawal, particularly of the more powerful drugs, may lead to anginal attacks with more pain or a decrease in exercise tolerance or heart attack. Therefore, reduction must be gradual as treatment progresses.

Generic name	Brand name	Dosage
glyceryl trinitrate	Angised, Coro-Nitro, Deponit, Minitran, Nitrocine, Nitrocontin Continus, Nitro-dur, Nitrolingual, Nitronal, Suscard, Sustac, Transiderm-Nitro	0.4–0.8 mg at onset of attack or prior to exertion (maximum 1.2 mg per attack)

Generic name	Brand name	Dosage
isosorbide dinitrate	Cedocard, Imtack, Isoket, Isordil, Soni-Slo, Sorbichew, Sorbid SA, Sorbitrate	Relief of angina attacks: 5–10 mg per dose Prevention of angina: 30–120 mg daily Left ventricular failure: 40–160 mg daily
isosorbide mononitrate	Elantan, Imdur, Ismo, Isotrate, MCR-50, Monit, Mono-Cedocard, Vascardin	40–120 mg daily

Table 5.2: Nitrates

Uses: angina pectoris, heart failure

When not to be used: heart attack, acute heart failure, low blood pressure, severe anaemia, head injury, stroke, aortic or mitral valve stenosis, low blood volume, cardiomyopathy (enlarged heart, heart failure, palpitations, embolism), constrictive pericarditis

Effects
  General: allergic reactions
  Cardiovascular: palpitations, rapid heart rate, slow heart rate, low blood pressure (particularly on standing)
  Central nervous system: headache, head injury, stroke
  Blood: anaemia
  Special senses: narrow-angle glaucoma

Strength level: 3 (1 if taken symptomatically)

CASE HISTORY

A woman aged 61 came for treatment with pain in her chest radiating to the jaw and left arm. The pain came on with exercise. An exercise ECG showed the effects of reduced blood flow to the heart and also brought on the pain.

She had a cough with green or yellow phlegm, was wheezy at times and had discomfort in the right side of her chest. She had hot flushes and woke at night feeling hot. She felt sad and depressed at such times. These chest symptoms came on after an emotional shock. She had had swollen ankles since the commencement of Istin medication.

Medication

Becotide inhaler: 2 puffs twice daily
Ventolin inhaler: 2 puffs 4 times daily
Istin: one daily
Transiderm nitro when needed for chest pain

Pulse: slippery, choppy and generally thin on the left side
Tongue: pale with some red patches centre, front and edges and stripping of the coat

Angina pectoris has several causes in Chinese medicine. These include: Qi Stagnation, stasis of Heart Blood, Cold Stagnation, Turbid Phlegm in the Chest, Deficiency of Qi, Yin or Yang.

In this case, I made a diagnosis of Phlegm Heat in the Lung, Turbid Phlegm in the Chest and Blood Deficiency. Treatment principles were: clear Heat and resolve Phlegm, Invigorate Yang, open the orifices, nourish and cool Blood.

It is important to determine what medication people are taking and why they are taking it. Below is an analysis of her prescribed drugs.

Drug	Type	Uses	Strength level
Becotide inhaler	Corticosteroid inhaler	Asthma	3
Ventolin inhaler	Bronchodilator inhaler	Asthma	2
Istin	Calcium channel blocker	Angina pectoris, hypertension	3
Transiderm nitro	Nitrate	Angina pectoris	1

The key drugs here are the Becotide and the Istin. The Transiderm nitro is already used symptomatically. Ventolin, although taken regularly in this case, can generally be moved easily to symptomatic treatment as the patient's symptoms subside. When considering Level 3 drugs, I generally deal with corticosteroids first, since they are very powerful and have a strong inhibiting action on the effectiveness of holistic treatment. This is true in whatever form they are used – oral, inhaled, rectal, skin applications and so on.

It is essential to treat first and wait for an improvement in the symptoms. Reduction in drug dosage can begin once the patient has decided on this and after an initial improvement in his/her condition.

I treated this patient with acupuncture and Chinese herbal medicine.

Acupuncture

P-6 Neiguan, **H-5** Tongli, **Ren-14** Juque, **Ren-17** Shanzhong, **LU-1** Zhongfu, **LU-5** Chize, **BL-13** Feishu, **BL-14** Jueyinshu, **ST-40** Fenglong

Chinese herbal medicine

Over the months of treatment, I used three main herbal formulae with this patient: firstly, a formula to resolve Phlegm, cool Heat and invigorate Yang; secondly, a formula to tonify Blood, Yin and Qi, together with herbs to move Qi; and, finally, a formula to harmonise the Qi.

Formula 1
Chuan Bei Mu *Bulbus Fritillariae Cirrhosae* 8 g
Tian Hua Fen *Radix Trichosanthis* 9 g
Gua Lou Zi *Semen Trichosanthis* 9 g
Fu Ling *Sclerotium Poriae Cocos* 6 g
Qing Pi *Pericarpium Citri Reticulatae Viride* 3 g
Jie Geng *Radix Platycodi Grandiflori* 3 g
Mai Men Dong *Tuber Ophiopogonis Japonici* 9 g
Xuan Shen *Radix Scrophulariae Ningpoensis* 5 g
Dan Shen *Radix Salviae Miltiorrhizae* 5 g
Dang Gui *Radix Angelicae Sinensis* 8 g
He Shou Wu *Radix Polygoni Multiflori* 6 g

Formula 2
Huang Qi *Radix Astragali* 18 g
He Shou Wu *Radix Polygoni Multiflori* 15 g
Dang Gui *Radix Angelicae Sinensis* 6 g
Shan Yao *Radix Dioscoreae Oppositae* 9 g

Dang Shen *Radix Codonopsis Pilosulae* 12 g
Huang Bai *Cortex Phellodendri* 5 g
Wu Yao *Radix Linderae Strychnifoliae* 3 g
Bei Sha Shen *Radix Glehniae Littoralis* 9 g
Mai Men Dong *Tuber Ophiopogonis Japonici* 9 g
Sang Ji Sheng *Ramus Loranthi seu Visci* 8 g
Fu Ling *Sclerotium Poriae Cocos* 6 g

Formula 3 (modified Xiao Yao San)
Chai Hu *Radix Bupleuri* 6 g
Bai Shao Yao *Radix Paeoniae Lactiflorae* 9 g
Dang Gui *Radix Angelicae Sinensis* 6 g
Bai Zhu *Rhizoma Atractylodis Macrocephalae* 8 g
Dan Shen *Radix Salviae Miltiorrhizae* 6 g
Fu Ling *Sclerotium Poriae Cocos* 6 g
Gan Cao *Radix GlycyrrhizaeUralensis* 3 g
Sheng Jiang *Cortex Zingiberis Officinalis Recens* 5 g
Da Zao *Fructus Zizyphi Jujubae* 3 g
Jie Geng *Radix Platycodi Grandiflori* 5 g
Xiang Fu *Rhizoma Cyperi Rotundi* 3 g

I usually use powdered herbs at a dosage of 2–4 g per day to be taken in hot water before food.

Outcome

The patient responded well to treatment, with an easing of her cough and phlegm. Her chest tightness settled and she felt well. These improvements allowed her to reduce her Becotide prescription. She reduced her dosage by 1 puff each time, so it took a couple of months to stop it altogether. After each reduction, we waited to see what symptoms might arise. Symptoms such as increased phlegm, more wheezing or tiredness can be expected when corticosteroid inhalers are reduced. It is helpful to proceed carefully and slowly. Any flare-up can then be treated and managed. When the flare-up settles and the patient is well again, it will be possible to reduce the dosage further.

When the Becotide was finally stopped, the patient moved on to reduce the Istin. Her chest pains had subsided by that stage, she felt well and she had no cough or phlegm. She reduced the Istin to one every second day. Her ankle swelling disappeared almost immediately. She experienced a mild recurrence of chest pains for a week or so after the Istin was reduced. We waited for this to settle and then she stopped the Istin a month later. By this time she did not need the Transiderm nitro and she was using the Ventolin inhaler only when necessary. This was only very occasionally for mild wheezing. She is now off all medication, is very well and active and comes for treatment every couple of months.

CHOLESTEROL-LOWERING DRUGS

These drugs reduce the levels of certain fats and fatty acids in the blood, particularly cholesterol. It is believed that an increased level of these substances can lead to early and more severe heart disease. However, the picture is more complicated, as there is increasing evidence that a low cholesterol level may be associated with certain chronic disease states. In addition, cholesterol has been somewhat demonised in the media and by the medical profession, despite the fact that it is a naturally occurring substance and is necessary for various vital functions within the body. With a marketing drive to sell low-fat milk and milk products as well as the recent development of drugs such as the statins (see below), the trend towards medicating for high cholesterol levels seems certain to continue.

Cholestyramine (colestyramine) and colestipol

Generic name	Brand name	Dosage
cholestyramine (colestyramine)	Questran, Questran Light	4–36 g daily
colestipol	Colestid	5–10 g daily (maximum 30 g daily)

Table 5.3:
Cholesterol-lowering drugs – cholestyramine (colestyramine) and colestipol

Uses: raised serum cholesterol

When not to be used: not in complete biliary obstruction

Cautions: if used long-term, Vitamin A, D and K supplements are recommended, because these drugs interfere with their absorption

Effects
General: weakness, severe allergic reactions, fatigue
Cardiovascular: chest pain
Respiratory: swelling of face and hands
Gastrointestinal: constipation, flatulence, indigestion, abdominal pain, nausea,

diarrhoea, raised liver enzymes, pancreatitis, hepatitis, jaundice, poor appetite, vomiting, high blood sugar, low blood sugar
Urogenital: impotence
Musculoskeletal: muscle pains, cramps and weakness, joint pains
Central nervous system: headache, pins and needles, dizziness, peripheral neuropathy causing weakness and numbness, vertigo
Psychological: insomnia
Blood: low platelet count (leading to bleeding into the skin, prolonged bleeding after injury and spontaneous bruising), anaemia
Skin: loss of head hair, itching, rash
Special senses: eye disorders

Strength level: 2

Statins

Generic name	Brand name	Dosage
atorvastatin	Lipitor	10–40 mg daily
fluvastatin	Lescol	20–40 mg daily
pravastatin	Lipostat, Pravachol	10–40 mg daily
simvastatin	Zocor	10–40 mg daily

Table 5.4: Cholesterol-lowering drugs – statins

Another statin, cerivastatin, was withdrawn in August 2001 when it was discovered that it causes muscle damage.

Uses: raised serum cholesterol

When not to be used: liver disease, those taking the oral contraceptive

Cautions: history of liver disease. Liver function tests must be performed before treatment has begun and repeated regularly during treatment.

This group of drugs can cause muscle damage that may be severe and even life-threatening. A creatine phosphokinase (CPK) level should be performed before treatment in anyone with kidney impairment, hypothyroidism, a personal or family history of inherited muscle disorders, previous muscle toxicity with one of these drugs and alcohol abuse. Patients over the age of 70 should be carefully assessed regarding the risk of muscle damage.

Effects

General: weakness, allergic reactions
Cardiovascular: chest pain
Respiratory: swelling of face and hands
Gastrointestinal: poor appetite, vomiting, constipation, flatulence, indigestion, abdominal pain, nausea, diarrhoea, raised liver enzymes, pancreatitis, hepatitis, jaundice, vomiting, low blood sugar, high blood sugar
Urogenital: impotence
Musculoskeletal: muscle pains and cramps, muscle inflammation, raised serum creatine phosphokinase (CPK), weakness and wasting of muscles
Central nervous system: headache, pins and needles, peripheral neuropathy causing weakness and numbness, dizziness
Psychological: insomnia
Skin: skin rashes, loss of head hair

Strength level: 2

Fibrates

Generic name	Brand name	Dosage
bezafibrate	Bezalip, Bezalip-Mono	400–600 mg daily
ciprofibrate	Modalim	100 mg daily
fenofibrate	Lipantil Micro 67, Lipantil Micro 200	200 mg daily
gemfibrozil	Gemfibrozil, Lopid	0.9–1.5 g daily

Table 5.5: Cholesterol-lowering drugs – fibrates

Uses: raised serum cholesterol

When not to be used: gallbladder disease or gallstones or a history of these, kidney or liver impairment, nephritic syndrome, alcoholism

Cautions: low serum protein levels (e.g. nephrotic syndrome), kidney impairment. Insulin requirements may change in patients with insulin-dependent diabetes mellitus.

Effects

General: fatigue
Gastrointestinal: mild gastrointestinal disturbances, gallstones, raised liver enzymes, raised serum creatine phosphokinase (CPK)

Urogenital: diminished libido
Musculoskeletal: muscle pain, weakness and wasting of muscles, rhabdomyolysis (muscle damage characterised by pain, weakness, tenderness, contractures, fever, rapid heart rate, nausea and vomiting; this may lead to kidney failure and cardiac arrest)
Central nervous system: headache, vertigo
Skin: skin reactions, sensitivity to light

Strength level: 2

Nicotinic acid

Generic name	Brand name	Dosage
acipmox	Olbetam	500–750 mg daily
nicotinic acid	–	100–200 mg 3 times daily, increasing to 1–2 g 3 times daily

Table 5.6: Cholesterol-lowering drugs – nicotinic acid

Uses: raised serum cholesterol

When not to be used: stomach or duodenal ulceration

Cautions: as the drug company literature states, 'evidence of clinical efficacy in the prevention of heart disease has not been established. The possible beneficial, and adverse, long-term consequences of some drugs used in the hyperlipidaemias are still the subject of scientific discussion.' This seems remarkable for a drug that is promoted as preventing heart disease.

Effects
  General: severe allergic reactions, malaise
  Respiratory: swelling of face and hands, wheezing
  Gastrointestinal: heartburn, indigestion, nausea, diarrhoea
  Central nervous system: headache
  Skin: sensation of heat, flushing, itching, rash, reddening of the skin, nettle rash

Strength level: 2

HOLISTIC MANAGEMENT

In conventional medicine, an attempt is made to control other risk factors before any patient embarks on drug treatment for raised cholesterol levels. These risk factors include smoking, female sex hormone treatment, alcohol use, excess weight, lack of exercise, diabetes mellitus and hypothyroidism. Because such treatment is considered to be long term, the patient's blood count and liver function have to be checked on at least two occasions before treatment begins. Cholesterol levels must also be checked at regular intervals. In animal experiments, some of these drugs in high doses produce liver tumours. This phenomenon has never been confirmed in humans, but clearly the drugs have a predilection to affect the liver.

These drugs are clearly powerful in their action and such treatment must not be undertaken lightly. I treated a 75-year-old patient some years ago when a survey was carried out locally, funded by a pharmaceutical company. The survey was into cholesterol levels and their drug treatment in people over the age of 70. I had treated the patient for some years for joint pains, intermittent insomnia and palpitations. He had been generally well during this time. However, when he began to take medication to lower his serum cholesterol (which was never very high), his whole energetic balance was disrupted. He became restless, with more disturbed sleep, and was generally overheated and suffered with sore eyes and headaches. He had more frequent palpitations and his blood pressure became high. He was then given medication for high blood pressure and, some four weeks later, had a stroke from which he never recovered.

When treating a patient who takes cholesterol-lowering drugs, it is helpful to run regular checks of serum cholesterol and other lipids. In practical terms, this means every couple of months or so. Holistic treatment is very effective at remedying the underlying imbalance that leads to raised levels in the first place. This, of course, needs to be accompanied by guidance on diet, exercise and, most importantly, relaxation. Excessive intake of sweet and greasy foods certainly leads to disturbances in cholesterol levels, but stress and psychological upset also play a major part. With holistic treatment, it is usually possible to withdraw cholesterol-lowering drugs in most patients after some months. It is more difficult to achieve normal levels of cholesterol in those people with a strong family history of high levels. Even then, however, holistic treatment will minimise any adverse effects of the medication.

6 ARTHRITIS

Prescribed drug use is common in all varieties of arthritis. Aspirin and non-steroidal anti-inflammatory drugs are given, despite there often being a lack of any degree of inflammation.[1] In such cases, paracetamol is equally effective.

Corticosteroids are injected locally into the joint or given systemically. Repeated injections weaken the joint and lead to further joint damage and deterioration. This is particularly true for weight-bearing joints. The drugs used in the treatment of arthritis (particularly rheumatoid arthritis) are listed in Table 6.1.

Treatment (mildest to strongest)	Strength level
Non-steroidal anti-inflammatory agents, including aspirin	2 (1 if taken symptomatically)
Sulphasalazine (sulfasalazine)	2
Gold, hydroxychloroquine and penicillamine	2
Corticosteroids	3
Immunosuppressants	3

Table 6.1: Drugs used in the treatment of arthritis

When treating patients taking drugs listed in Table 6.1, it is important, as usual, to wait for an initial improvement in the patient's condition and symptoms. Focus on one drug at a time and complete its reduction and withdrawal before moving onto another. Withdrawal symptoms mainly centre on the joints, with a flare-up of swelling, pain and stiffness. It is helpful to begin with corticosteroids, then to move on to second-line agents such as gold, chloroquine and its relatives and penicillamine before dealing with the non-steroidal anti-inflammatory drugs (NSAIDs). In this way, the weaker drugs can support the patient and be used to alleviate pain as treatment progresses. When the second-line agents are withdrawn in cases of rheumatoid arthritis, some constitutional symptoms may appear such as fever, poor appetite, tiredness and so on.

In rheumatoid arthritis, which is an example of a deep, degenerative disease of the immune system, treatment will necessarily be prolonged and so there is plenty of time to reduce dosage. Corticosteroids are discussed in more detail on page 51.

NON-STEROIDAL ANTI-INFLAMMATORY DRUGS (NSAIDS)

Non-steroidal anti-inflammatory drugs are commonly used in the treatment of arthritis because they have an effect on inflammation and also relieve pain. They are of similar effectiveness to paracetamol in their ability to ease pain. Some NSAIDs may be given for painful periods, back pain or acute strains and sprains. As a group, they are similar in action to aspirin and are in common use. They are acidic in nature, have powerful effects on the gastrointestinal tract and lead to analgesic nephropathy.[36]

Generic name	Brand name	Dosage
aceclofenac	Preservex	200 mg daily
acemetacin	Emflex	120–180 mg daily
aspirin[37]	Anadin, Angettes, Ascriptin, Aspav, Aspro, Caprin, Codis, Cox Dispersible, Disprin, Dristan, Equagesic, Nu-Seals, Resprin (Suppositories), Veganin	Pain/fever: 300–900 mg per dose Prevention of blood clots: 75–300 mg daily
azapropazone	Rheumox	1.2 g daily
benorylate (benorilate)	Benoral, Benorilate	4–8 g daily
diclofenac	Arthrotec*, Cataflam, Diclomax SR, Diclomel, Difene, Fenac, Flexagen, Fortfen, Motefine, Motifene, Panamor, Rhumalgan, Sodiclo, Volraman, Voltarol, Vologen, Voltaren	75–150 mg daily
diflusinal	Dolobid	1 g daily
etodolac	Lodine SR	600 mg daily
felbinac	Traxam	25 g daily maximum

fenbufen	Lederfen, Fenbuzip	900 mg daily Not for children
fenoprofen	Fenopron, Nalfon, Progesic	300–600 mg 3–4 times daily
flurbiprofen	Ansaid, Froben, Ocufen	100–300 mg daily
ibuprofen	Aches-N-Pain, Actiprofen, ACT-3, Advil, Antiflam, Apsifen, Arthrofen, Brufen, Bufigen, Codafen*, Cuprofen, Ebufac, Fenbid, Haltran, IBU, Ibufac, Ibufem, Ibugel, Ibuleve, Inoven, Inza, Junifen, Lidifen Melfen, Motrin, Novaprin, Nuprin, Nurofen, Paxofen, Rafen, Ranfen, Solfen, Trendar, Vicoprofen*	Pain relief: 600 mg–1.8 g daily Children: usually 20 mg/kg daily Maximum: 500 mg daily for those less than 30 kg Arthritis: 1.2–2.4 g daily
indomethacin (indometacin)	Acuflex, Articulen, Artracin, Arthrexin, Cidomel, Cox, Flamaret, Flexin Continus, Imbrilon, Indameth, Indocid, Indocin, Indoflex, Indolar, Indomax, Indomed, Indomod, Hicin, Maximet, Mobilan, Nisaid, Rheumacin LA, Slo-Indo	50–200 mg daily
ketoprofen	Alrheumat, Fenoket, Ketocid, Ketovail, Ketozip, Larafen, Orudis, Oruvail, Rhodis	150–200 mg daily
mefenamic acid	Dysman, Mefic, Meflam, Opustan, Ponalgic, Ponmel, Ponstan, Ponstel	1.5 mg daily
nabumetone	Relafen, Relifex, Relisan	0.5–1 g daily

naproxen	Acusprain, Aleve, Anaprox, Arthrosin, Arthroxen, Inza, Laraflex, Napmel, Napratec*, Naprelan, Naprosyn, Naprogesic, Nycopren, Prosaid, Proxen, Synflex, Timpron, Traumox, Valrox	Mild to moderate pain, menstrual cramps: 250 mg 3–4 times daily Muscular pain and arthritis: 500–1,250 mg daily Gout: 250 mg 3 times daily
nimesulide	Aulin, Mesulid	1–2 twice daily
phenylbutazone	Azolid, Butacote, Butatab, Butazolidin	100 mg 2–3 times daily
piroxicam	Candyl, Feldene, Fensaid, Flamatrol, Kentene, Larapram, Mobilis, Pericam Piroflam, Pirox, Pirozip, Roxicam, Xycam	1–40 mg daily
rofecoxib	Vioxx	12.5–25 mg daily
sulindac	Aclin, Apo-Sulin, Clinoril, Clusinol, R-Flex, Saldac	200 mg twice daily
tenoxicam	Mobiflex, Tilcotil	20 mg daily
tiaprofenic acid	Surgam	600 mg daily
tolmetin	Tolectin	600–1,800 mg daily

Table 6.1: Non-steroidal anti-inflammatory drugs (NSAIDs)

Uses: arthritis, mild to moderate pain, fever, dysmenorrhoea, muscle strain, migraine

When not to be used: stomach or duodenal ulcers, ulcerative colitis, blood disorders, liver or kidney impairment.

Suppositories should not be used in those with inflammation of the anus, rectum or sigmoid colon.

Many NSAIDs cause liver damage, as evidenced by their effect of raised liver enzymes. Nimesulide is under examination at the time of writing (September 2002) as being more hazardous. It is currently suspended from use in Finland, Spain and Turkey.

Cautions: wheezing can be brought on in people with asthma or allergies.

People with impaired hearing should have regular tests of hearing function. Eye examinations should be done if visual disturbances occur. All patients receiving long-term treatment should be regularly monitored by means of kidney and liver function tests and blood counts.

Some patients may develop severe kidney disease. Urinary system symptoms of painful urination, cystitis, blood in the urine, nephritis and nephrotic syndrome may occur. Some patients may need dialysis and treatment with corticosteroids. Those who are particularly liable to these effects include the elderly, those taking diuretics and those with kidney or liver impairment and heart failure.

Raised liver enzymes are seen in 15% of patients. The drugs must be stopped if liver enzyme tests worsen, as severe liver reactions, including jaundice and death, have occurred.

Care must be taken in those with high blood pressure and impaired function of the heart, because some people develop oedema when on these drugs.

Effects
>   *General:* allergic reactions
>   *Cardiovascular:* oedema, heart failure, fluid retention
>   *Respiratory:* swelling of face and hands, wheezing, cough, breathlessness
>   *Gastrointestinal:* nausea, diarrhoea, stomach or duodenal ulcers, vomiting blood, raised liver enzymes, liver damage, indigestion
>   *Urogenital:* impaired kidney function, blood in urine, cloudy urine, loin pain, painful urination, frequent urination, nocturnal urination, incontinence
>   *Central nervous system:* headache, dizziness, vertigo, aseptic meningitis causing fever, neck stiffness and sensitivity to light
>   *Blood: low platelet count* leading to bleeding into the skin, prolonged bleeding after injury and spontaneous bruising
>   *Skin:* sensitivity to light, Stevens-Johnson syndrome (fever, blistering of mouth, throat, anus and eyes), toxic epidermal necrolysis (life-threatening condition where the skin peels off in sheets leaving areas stripped of skin)
>   *Special senses:* blurred vision, hearing disturbances, tinnitus, eye changes

Strength level: 2

GOLD

This is a 'second-line' drug for rheumatoid arthritis and does not produce a full response until after 4–6 months of treatment. It may be given by injection or orally.

Generic name	Brand name	Dosage
auranofin	Ridaura	6–9 mg daily

Table 6.2: Gold

Uses: rheumatoid arthritis, arthritis of psoriasis, juvenile arthritis

When not to be used: pulmonary fibrosis, necrotising enterocolitis, exfoliative dermatitis (severe skin condition characterised by fever, redness, itching and scaling of skin), severe blood diseases, severe kidney or liver disease, systemic lupus erythematosus

Cautions: kidney or liver impairment, inflammatory bowel disease, rash, history of bone marrow depression.

Full blood count and urinary analysis for protein must be checked before treatment begins and monthly.

People who have symptoms such as rash, itching, sore mouth or metallic taste in the mouth must be closely monitored, as the drug may have to be reduced in dosage or withdrawn. People should be warned to report symptoms such as itching, rash, metallic taste in the mouth, sore throat or tongue, mouth ulceration, easy bruising, bleeding into the skin, nose bleeds, bleeding gums, heavy periods or diarrhoea.

This drug can damage a developing foetus, so women must avoid becoming pregnant during treatment and for at least six months after treatment has ended.

Effects
Cardiovascular: oedema
Respiratory: breathlessness, dry cough
Gastrointestinal: diarrhoea, nausea, abdominal pain, diarrhoea with bleeding and mucus, taste in the mouth usually metallic, sore mouth, raised liver enzymes
Urogenital: nephrotic syndrome, blood in urine, kidney impairment
Central nervous system: headaches, dizziness, peripheral neuropathy causing weakness and numbness
Blood: reduction in white blood cell count that may lead to increased infections,

reduction in numbers of granulocytes (type of white blood cell), *low platelet count* leading to bleeding into the skin, prolonged bleeding after injury and spontaneous bruising, *severe acute reduction in numbers of neutrophils* (type of white blood cell) leading to severe bacterial infections that are usually fatal, *increase in numbers of eosinophils* (type of white blood cell) usually denoting allergic reaction, *reduction in numbers of red and white blood cells and platelets* leading to anaemia, increased risk of infection and spontaneous bruising/bleeding

Skin: rashes with itching, loss of head hair, exfoliative dermatitis (severe skin condition characterised by fever, redness, itching and scaling of skin)

Strength level: 2

PENICILLAMINE

This is a 'second-line' drug for rheumatoid arthritis and does not produce a full response until after 4–6 months of treatment. The drug should be stopped if there is no improvement after a year of treatment. More people can tolerate penicillamine than gold, but people frequently experience many side-effects.

Generic name	Brand name	Dosage
penicillamine	Distamine, Pendramine	125–250 mg daily, increasing to 500–750 mg over 6–12 months

Table 6.3: Penicillamine

Uses: rheumatoid arthritis

When not to be used: agranulocytosis, persistent protein in the urine, systemic lupus erythematosus

Cautions: full blood count, platelet counts and kidney function tests must be done before treatment and at regular intervals (usually monthly). Particular attention must be given to those with kidney impairment.

Effects
   General: fever, Goodpasture's syndrome, Pseudoxanthoma elasticum
   Gastrointestinal: nausea, poor appetite, loss of taste
   Urogenital: protein in urine, blood in urine, nephrotic syndrome, kidney impairment
   Musculoskeletal: systemic lupus erythematosus, myasthenia gravis, rheumatoid arthritis

Blood: low platelet count leading to bleeding into the skin, prolonged bleeding after injury and spontaneous bruising, *severe acute reduction in numbers of neutrophils* (type of white blood cell) leading to severe bacterial infections that are usually fatal, *reduction in numbers of red and white blood cells and platelets* leading to anaemia, increased risk of infection and bleeding into the skin, prolonged bleeding after injury and spontaneous bruising, *anaemia* due to destruction of red blood cells
Skin: rash, pemphigus, Stevens-Johnson syndrome (fever, blistering of mouth, throat, anus and eyes), epidermolysis bullosa (blistering and scarring of skin, mouth and throat), dermatomyositis

Strength level: 2

HYDROXYCHLOROQUINE

This is a 'second-line' drug with similar uses and effects to gold and penicillamine. It has a propensity to cause eye damage.

Generic name	Brand name	Dosage
hydroxy-chloroquine	Plaquenil	200–400 mg daily

Table 6.4: Hydroxychloroquine

Uses: rheumatoid arthritis, systemic lupus erthyematosus

When not to be used: eye disease affecting the macula

Cautions: disorders of liver, kidney, nervous system, blood or digestive system, porphyria; anyone taking drugs that affect the liver or kidneys.

All patients should have an eye examination before treatment and at least every six months during treatment. This drug must be stopped immediately if eye symptoms develop. Care particularly needs to be taken if the patient is also taking drugs that affect the eyes or skin.

Serum hydroxychloroquine levels should be performed in people with marked liver or kidney impairment. Regular blood counts are recommended.

Effects
Cardiovascular: cardiomyopathy (enlarged heart, heart failure, palpitations, embolism)

Gastrointestinal: nausea, diarrhoea, poor appetite, abdominal cramps, vomiting, raised liver enzymes, liver failure
Musculoskeletal: muscle weakness, weakness and wasting of muscles
Central nervous system: vertigo, headache, convulsions, peripheral neuropathy causing weakness and numbness
Psychological: emotional upsets, psychosis, nervousness
Blood: bone marrow depression
Skin: rashes, colour changes in skin and lining of mouth, white hair, loss of head hair, exfoliative dermatitis (severe skin condition characterised by fever, redness, itching and scaling of skin), psoriasis, changes in pigmentation
Special senses: retinal and corneal damage, visual symptoms such as reduced field of vision, haloes, blurring and sensitivity to light, tinnitus, nerve deafness

Strength level: 2

CORTICOSTEROIDS

These are hormones produced by the adrenal glands and have many functions concerned with responses to shock, infection and stressful situations, as well as having a role in carbohydrate metabolism.

Clinically, they are used primarily for their anti-inflammatory actions.

Oral corticosteroids

Generic name	Brand name	Dosage
betamethasone	Betnelan, Betnesol	0.5–5 mg daily
cortisone	Cortelan, Cortisyl	25–37.5 mg daily
deflazacort	Calcort	3–18 mg daily
dexamethasone	Decadron, Oradexon	0.5–10 mg daily
fludrocortisone	Florinef	50–300 mcg daily
hydrocortisone	Cortef, Hydrocortone, Hysone, Solu-Cortef	20–30 mg daily
methyl prednisolone	A-methaPred, Medrol, Medrone, Solu-Medrol, Solu-Medrone	2–40 mg daily

prednisolone	Codelsol, Deltacortril, Deltasolone, Deltastab, Hydeltrasol, Key-Pred SP, Nor Pred-S, Panafcortelone, Pedate S Prednis, Precortisyl, Precortisyl Forte, Prednesol, Solone	2.5–15 mg daily (higher doses are sometimes seen)

Table 6.5: Corticosteroids – oral

Uses: suppresses the symptoms of inflammation and allergy and so are used in autoimmune diseases such as rheumatoid arthritis, systemic lupus erythematosus, scleroderma, polyarteritis nodosa, nephritis (inflammation of the kidney), inflammatory bowel disease, eczema, psoriasis and asthma. Also used in some cancer treatments and in organ transplantation. It is common nowadays to see oral corticosteroids used for infections such as bronchitis, where there is a lot of phlegm and perhaps some wheezing. They will be prescribed together with antibiotics and perhaps a bronchodilator inhaler.

Cortisone, fludrocortisone and hydrocortisone are used in underactivity of the adrenal cortex (Addison's disease) and are classified as strength Level 5 (see page22).

When not to be used: those receiving live virus vaccination

Cautions: tuberculosis or history of tuberculosis

Effects
  General: this group of drugs leads to marked changes in metabolism, particularly of carbohydrates and protein. There will be retention of sodium and loss of potassium, leading to fluid retention. Calcium is lost from the body, as is protein. Allergic reactions, malaise.
  Cardiovascular: heart failure, rupture of heart muscle, thrombosis, high blood pressure, fluid retention
  Respiratory: oedema of face and upper body
  Gastrointestinal: stomach or duodenal ulcer, perforated ulcer, pancreatitis, abdominal distension, ulcerated oesophagus, indigestion, thrush in the oesophagus, weight gain, increased appetite, nausea
  Central nervous system: convulsions, vertigo, headache
  Endocrine: development of Cushingoid state, suppression of growth in children, decreased carbohydrate tolerance, diabetes mellitus, need for increased dosages of insulin or oral hypoglycaemic agents in diabetics

Women's health: menstrual irregularities, no periods

Psychological: it is extremely common to see an elevated mood in patients who take corticosteroids. Euphoria is common. People feel hot, sweaty and more energetic and have difficulty sleeping. In severe cases, people can become manic and occasionally psychotic.

Blood: increase in number of white blood cells

Skin: delayed wound healing, thin fragile skin, petechiae and ecchymoses, redness, stretch marks, telangiectasis, acne, allergic dermatitis, nettle rash, hair growth

Special senses: cataracts, glaucoma, thinning of cornea or sclera, worsening of eye infections (particularly viral), exophthalmos, visual loss

Strength level: 3 (5 if used in cancer treatment, organ transplantation or Addison's disease)

Inhaled corticosteroids

Generic name	Brand name	Dosage
beclomethasone (beclometasone)	AeroBec, Asmabec Clickhaler, BDP Spacehaler, Beclazone, Becloforte, Becodisks, Beconase, Becotide, Filair, Qvar, Ventide*	1–2 puffs 3–4 times daily, depending on precise drug used
budesonide	Pulmicort, Pulmicort LS, Pulmicort Turbohaler	1–2 puffs 3–4 times daily
fluticasone	Flixotide, Seretide*	1–2 puffs 3–4 times daily

Table 6.6: Corticosteroids – inhaled

Uses: asthma

Inhaled corticosteroids are also prescribed in cases of acute infective bronchitis (along with antibiotics), emphysema and other cases of chronic lung disease.

When not to be used: hypersensitivity and allergy

Cautions: tuberculosis and history of tuberculosis

Effects (inhaled corticosteroids have much less powerful effects than the oral forms)
General: growth retardation definitely occurs with inhaled corticosteroids, although this is never listed in the literature

Respiratory: wheezing, hoarseness, throat irritation
Gastrointestinal: thrush in the mouth and throat
Special senses: cataracts

Strength level: 3

Corticosteroids for skin use

These corticosteroids are used in the treatment of a wide range of skin disorders, including eczema and psoriasis (although their use in psoriasis is not generally recommended as good practice). They are divided into different categories, according to their strength.

Generic name	Brand name	Dosage
alcomethasone	Modrasone	The lowest dosage that will produce an acceptable result should be used
fluocinolone	Synalar 1:10	
hydrocortisone	Actinac*, Alphaderm*, Alphosyl HC*, Barquinol HC*, Calmurid HC*, Canesten HC*, Carbocort*, Cobadex*, Daktacort*, Dioderm, Econacort*, Eczederm HC*, Efcortelan, Epifoam*, Eurax-Hydro-cortisone*, Framycort*, Fucidin H*, Genticin HC*, Gregoderm*, Hydrocal*, Hydrocortistab, Hydro-cortisyl, Mildison, Nystaform HC*, Quinocort*, Quino-derm with Hydrocortisone*, Sential*, Tarcartin*, Terra-Cortril, Terra-Cortril Nystatin*, Timodine*, Tricicatrin*, Vioform-Hydrocortisone*	
methyl-prednisolone	Medrone*, Neo-Medrone*	

Table 6.7: Mildly potent corticosteroids for skin use

Generic name	Brand name	Dosage
clobetasone	Eumovate, Trimovate*	The lowest dosage that will produce an acceptable result should be used
desoxymethasone (desoximetasone)	Stiedex LP, Stiedex LP N*	
fluocinolone	Synalar 1:4	
fluocortolone	Ultradil, Ultralanum	
flurandrenolone (fludroxycortide)	Haelan, Haelan Tape, Haelan-X, Haelan-C*	
hydrocortisone	Alphaderm*, Calmurid HC*	

Table 6.8: Moderately potent corticosteroids for skin use

Generic name	Brand name	Dosage
beclomethasone (beclometasone)	Propaderm, Propaderm A*	The lowest dosage that will produce an acceptable result should be used
betamethasone	Betnovate, Betnovate C*, Betnovate N*, Betnovate RD, Diprosalic*, Diprosone, Fucibet*, Lotriderm*	
budesonide	Preferid	
desoxymethasone (desoximetasone)	Stiedex	
diflucortolone	Nerisone	
fluclorolone	Topilar	
fluocinolone	Synalar, Synalar Gel, Synalar C*, Synalar N*	
fluocinonide	Metosyn	
hydrocortisone 17-butyrate	Locoid, Locoid C*	
triamcinolone	Adcortyl, Adcortyl with Graneodin*, Aureocort*, Ledercort, Nystadermal*, Pevaryl TC*, Tri-Adcortyl*	

Table 6.9: Potent corticosteroids for skin use

Generic name	Brand name	Dosage
clobetasol	Dermovate, Dermovate NN*	The lowest dosage that will produce an acceptable result should be used
diflucortolone	Nerisone Forte, Halciderm	

Table 6.10: Very potent corticosteroids for skin use

Uses: inflammatory skin conditions, e.g. eczema

When not to be used: infective skin conditions (although combinations of corticosteroids plus anti-bacterial or anti-fungal preparations may be given), acne rosacea, acne vulgaris

Cautions: extreme care must be taken in babies and children and on sensitive areas (e.g. face and eyes)

Effects
    General: suppression of adrenal function, especially in children and babies
    Skin: dermatitis, acne, worsening of rosacea, wrinkling and thinning of skin, stretch marks, dilatation of blood vessels, susceptibility to injury, delayed wound healing, worsening of ulceration, loss of or increased pigmentation, nettle rash, sensitivity to light; psoriasis may worsen and develop into pustular form

Strength level: 3

HOLISTIC MANAGEMENT OF CORTICOSTEROIDS

Corticosteroids are extremely powerful drugs, as evidenced by the list of their effects. The oral forms are the strongest in their effect. They will produce a situation similar to Cushing's syndrome – overactivity of the adrenal cortex – at moderate dosages. For example, more than 7.5 mg of prednisolone daily will always lead to many 'cushingoid' effects. They are powerful suppressants of inflammation and rapidly antidote treatment with holistic medicine. However, corticosteroids in any form – inhaler, skin application, nasal spray, enema and so on – will all have powerful effects.

Oral corticosteroids must never be stopped suddenly, as they suppress adrenal function and it takes some time for the adrenal glands to recover when the dosage of corticosteroids is reduced. With sudden and rapid reduction in dosage, there is a risk of overwhelming infection and collapse of blood pressure leading to shock – the symptoms of Addison's disease (underactivity of the adrenal cortex). In selected cases, it is possible to reduce or even stop corticosteroids, but this must be done slowly and only after careful consideration of:

- dose
- duration of the medication
- the condition for which it was given
- other treatment
- the patient's energetic state

Corticosteroids are very depleting and people who take them for a long time are generally in a weakened state when they present for treatment. Treatment will be slow and difficult if the use of corticosteroids has been long term, the patient's energy is weak and the clinical picture unclear. Diagnosis and treatment are more straightforward if the use of corticosteroids has been long term yet the person's energy is stronger and the clinical picture is clear. You may have to treat more often than usual, because of the powerful effects of the corticosteroids. Some homoeopaths use more frequent administration of low-potency remedies. However, holistic treatment can still be effective 'through' the drug.

The case can be taken as usual and treatment initiated if the use of corticosteroids is not current. It is common for people who have had these drugs in the past to be more difficult to treat. Treatment tends to be longer and aggravations are more severe. However, such patients can usually be treated quite successfully. The same rules apply, whether the drug is administered orally, inhaled, applied to the skin, used as an enema, etc.

Treat the patient until an improvement occurs. Bear in mind the original diagnosis, since exacerbations may be potentially serious. Reduce the dose slowly, e.g. if 6 mg of prednisolone is being taken daily in a case of asthma, the reduction would be around 1 mg every three to four weeks. It should certainly be no quicker than this.

Corticosteroids differ in their strength of action. The equivalents to 1 mg of prednisolone are:

- 0.12 mg betamethasone
- 0.5 mg cortisone
- 0.15 mg dexamethasone
- 0.4 mg hydrocortisone
- 0.8 mg methylprednisolone
- 0.8 mg triamcinolone

Encourage people to use other drugs they may be taking, such as bronchodilators in asthma, non-steroidal anti-inflammatory drugs in rheumatoid arthritis and so on. These will support the patient whilst the powerful corticosteroids are reduced. It is usually possible to begin reducing the less powerful drugs once the corticosteroids are eventually stopped.

I am currently treating a woman aged 77 who was given corticosteroids because of stiff shoulders and tiredness. She was taking 5 mg of Deltacortril daily. Even at that dosage, she experienced symptoms of weight gain, increased appetite and restless sleep. After some weeks of treatment, she reduced her medication to 5 mg and 2.5 mg on alternate days (this is the equivalent of reducing by 1.25 mg each day). She felt tired for several days after the reduction but otherwise well. One month later, she reduced to 2.5 mg daily. Again, she felt tired, with some return of stiffness in her shoulders. We waited for two months for these symptoms to subside and for further holistic treatment to be applied before reducing further. The next reduction in dosage was to take 2.5 mg daily for two days, nothing for the third day and then this pattern was repeated. This is equivalent to a dosage reduction of 0.83 mg daily. In this way, the reduction is slow and manageable. There was always an increase in tiredness for several days after each reduction, as you would expect when a stimulant drug is decreased in dosage. It took over six months for her to come off the corticosteroids completely.

CASE HISTORY

A woman of 30 presented for treatment with generalised pains in the joints. She had been involved in a road traffic accident some three months previously when she had sustained marked bruising over her right hypochondrium and abdominal wall from the safety belt. Some four weeks after the accident, she developed pains in the chest (which were aggravated by breathing), stiffness in the muscles and joints, hot swellings of the joints, nausea, fever, night sweats and general malaise and tiredness.

Her symptoms worsened to the point where she could hardly move and she had to be admitted to hospital. After some days, a diagnosis of polyarteritis nodosa[38] was made and she was given:

- prednisolone – 100 mg daily
- azathioprine – 125 mg daily

Her symptoms quickly improved and, at the time of her consultation with me, she had some residual tightness and discomfort in the chest, weakness in the legs and hot and swollen wrists. Her appetite was normal now and she slept well. Her dosage of prednisolone had been reduced to 60 mg daily. She came for treatment because she wanted relief of her symptoms and to come off her drugs. Her consultant had specifically told her that the drugs had no side-effects. However, she had met people who had taken corticosteroids long term and realised that she was likely to develop problems; particularly at the dosage that she had been prescribed.

The dosage of corticosteroids reflects the strength of inflammation in this case. As she had been on the medication for some two months now, it was not sensible to reduce quickly. I impressed on her that the appropriate time to start drug reduction would be when she started to improve. If she reduced them too soon, then the original clinical picture might return.

In terms of Chinese medicine, her diagnosis was DampHeat Stagnation, which was confirmed by a pulse quality that was full and slippery. Her tongue was pale and swollen, which is contradictory, as it would be expected to be red with a thick, yellow greasy coat. This was because of the effect of the corticosteroids. The accident was clearly the trigger, because of damage to the Blood, particularly Liver Blood, given the site of the injury. A predisposing cause was taking the oral contraceptive, which tends to lead to Blood disturbances, particularly Stagnation. Also, she had a history of a kidney 'infection' (when aged 7), which had necessitated hospital admission. Prior to and after the car accident, she was under a lot of emotional strain at home.

I gave her an acupuncture treatment and five packets of herbs to release the Stagnation and protect the Blood. She returned some two weeks later and told me that, after her last visit, she had decided to stop the prescribed drugs and had flushed them down the toilet! She felt very shaky and nauseous for a week, but this had then settled down. She now had very few symptoms, which included some aching in her neck and wrists. Her general weakness had subsided and there were no swellings.

Over the course of the next few months, I concentrated on correcting her underlying Kidney and Blood imbalances. After six months of treatment, she was well with no problems.

This case illustrates several important points. Her initial reaction to the injury illustrated a pre-existing susceptibility at a fairly deep level. However, the strong nature of her symptoms, the acute onset and her rapid response to treatment reveal a basically strong constitution. This was responsible for her clearly taking charge of her medication. Two months of medication is not long enough to lead to significant suppression of adrenal function and, if the holistic treatment is correct, there will be little in the way of flare-up.

This brings me to the question of the energetic action of corticosteroids. There is some discussion as to whether they are Cold or Hot in nature, as they are commonly used for inflammatory conditions. The key is to look at what happens if the body does not produce its own supply of corticosteroids or if corticosteroids (prescribed long-term) are withdrawn rapidly. The clinical appearance is that of Addison's disease. There is low blood pressure, low temperature, general slowing of the body functions and eventually coma and death. This corresponds to a collapse of the Yang picture in Chinese medicine and so corticosteroids would be the counterpart of a Rescue Yang formula.

They are Hot in nature and primarily affect the Lung, Spleen and Kidney Yang. They are strongly dispersing and release Stagnation syndromes such as Bi Syndrome. They are also toxic. They will rescue the Yang Deficiency with Water Overflowing of severe cardiac insufficiency. Over time, they will lead to depletion of Blood and Yin, especially of the Liver and Kidney. In the acute phase, because the Heat is due to Stagnation, the clinical symptoms and signs of Heat will disappear. This is why this woman's tongue was pale rather than the expected red with a thick yellow coat. In long-term use, Heat will be much more evident as the fluids become damaged.

Since these drugs are Hot and strongly moving, they disperse the Yang Qi of the Lung, Spleen and Kidney. This explains the typical side-effects of oedema, especially of the upper and middle parts of the body. The Lung is responsible for the water passages through its dispersing and descending function and the Spleen transforms and transports. Interference with these two organs leads to oedema.

There will be increased appetite due to Stomach Heat, wasting of the limbs due to the damage to body fluids and muscles, diabetes mellitus can develop as the Yin is consumed and heating of the Heart can lead to mental disturbances and psychotic manifestations in some. The effect on Lung Yang explains the relief obtained from wheezing in asthma. Long term, of course, there will be Kidney Yin and Yang Deficiency as this organ is weakened.

Other case histories involving the use of corticosteroids are described on pages 69 and 159.

Note

[1] There are a wide range of, so-called, autoimmune diseases, where the immune system attacks the body's own tissues. Rheumatoid arthritis is the most common one to affect the joints, but there are others, including polyarteritis nodosa.

7 ASTHMA

Asthma is very common. It is seen in both children and adults and may have an allergic component, particularly in younger patients. The basis of conventional treatment is with drugs, although patients may also be given advice about exercise and breathing.

There is an increasing tendency to treat asthma 'aggressively' – that is, to start treatment earlier, for milder cases, and to use corticosteroid inhalers at the beginning of treatment rather than waiting to see the effect of bronchodilators. Other diseases with wheezing, such as chronic bronchitis and emphysema, are also sometimes treated with these drugs but with limited results. Although inhaled drugs cause less general side-effects than if they were taken orally, their effect on the lung tends to be more insidious and, of course, still suppressive.

The first-line treatment of asthma and wheezing is with a bronchodilator, of which there are several types available. These drugs stimulate the lungs and heart and, over time, lead to weakness of these organs. Therefore, the longer patients have taken these drugs, the more likely there is to be chronic damage. In fact, bronchodilators in the past, such as ephedrine and adrenaline (epinephrine), have led to deaths. There is currently some belief, even in orthodox circles, that increasing asthma deaths now may be linked to these agents, particularly fenoterol. In 1990, fenoterol was withdrawn from the market in New Zealand and Australia. A recent survey[1] reported that the risk of death in asthma was significantly greater in those who have received more than one prescription for bronchodilators in the previous 12 months. This suggests, as have previous studies, that increased use of bronchodilators leads to more problems for people because of their effect on cardiac and lung function.

Treatment (mildest to strongest)	Strength level
Sodium cromoglycate (sodium cromoglicate)	2

Bronchodilators
    inhaled
    nebulised
    oral
	2

Corticosteroid
    inhaled (see page 53)
    oral (see page 51)
    injected
	3

Table 7.1: Drug treatment of asthma

SODIUM CROMOGLYCATE AND RELATED DRUGS

Sodium cromoglycate (sodium cromoglicate) is used to prevent attacks in allergic asthma, although it is not understood how it works and some people who would be expected to respond do not. It is taken regularly. It is not considered to be effective in an acute attack. My experience is that some people gain relief from wheezing by taking a dose of sodium cromoglycate at the time of the attack. It would therefore seem to have similar energetic effects to the bronchodilators.

Generic name	Brand name	Dosage
nedocromil	Tilade	Inhaler – 2 puffs 4 times daily
sodium cromoglycate (sodium cromoglicate)	Aerocrom*, Cromogen, Intal	Inhaler – 2 puffs 4 times daily

Table 7.2:
Sodium cromoglycate (sodium cromoglicate) and related drugs

Uses: asthma

Effects
    Respiratory: throat irritation, cough, wheezing

Strength level: 2

BETA-ADRENOCEPTOR STIMULANTS

Beta-adrenoceptor stimulants are a commonly prescribed group of drugs that relieve wheezing in asthma. They stimulate receptors in the lung that are affected by adrenaline- (epinephrine-) like substances. This explains the common side-effects of agitation, restlessness, rapid pulse and tremor.

They may also be given to patients with chronic lung disease, such as chronic bronchitis or emphysema, with limited success. They are usually given in inhaled form, although some are available orally. In more severe cases, they may be applied by nebuliser. They are frequently given together with corticosteroids, usually in inhaled form, but occasionally orally.

Generic name	Brand name	Dosage
bambuterol	Bambec	10–20 mg daily
eformoterol (formoterol)	Foradil, Oxis	1–2 puffs once or twice daily
ephedrine[2]	–	Adults: 15–60 mg 3 times daily
fenoterol	Berotec, Duovent*	1–2 puffs 1–3 times daily Children aged 6–12: 1 puff 1–3 times daily
orciprenaline	Alupent	1–2 puffs every 30 minutes if necessary (maximum of 12 puffs daily)
pirbuterol	Maxair	2 puffs 3–4 times daily (maximum of 12 puffs daily)
reproterol	Bronchodil	1–2 puffs 3 times daily Children aged 6–12: 1 puff 3 times daily
salbutamol (albuterol)	Aerocrom*, Aerolin, Airomir, Asmasal Clickhaler, Asmaven, Combivent*, Maxivent, Proventil, Salamol, Salbulin, Ventide*, Ventodisks, Ventolin, Volmax	Inhaler: 1–2 puffs 3–4 times daily Orally: 4 mg 3 times daily

salmeterol	Seretide*, Serevent	2–4 puffs twice daily Children over 4 years: 1 puff twice daily
terbutaline	Bricanyl, Monovent	Inhaler: 1–2 puffs 3–4 times daily Orally: 2.5–5 mg 3 times daily
tulobuterol	Respacal	2 mg twice or 3 times daily

Table 7.3: Beta-adrenoceptor stimulants

Uses: asthma

Cautions: hyperthyroidism, heart failure, angina, palpitations, hypertension, diabetes mellitus, kidney disease (over 50% of the drug is excreted by the kidney).

Care should also be exercised if taken with drugs that are stimulating in nature, such as monoamine oxidase inhibitor antidepressants, tricyclic antidepressants or sympathomimetic agents.

These drugs prolong pregnancy and slow down labour.

Effects
> *General:* weakness, collapse
> *Cardiovascular:* palpitations, low blood pressure, hot extremities, flushing, rapid heart rate
> *Respiratory:* oedema of face and upper body, wheezing
> *Gastrointestinal:* dry mouth, cough, mouth and throat irritation, stomach upset
> *Urogenital:* difficult urination
> *Musculoskeletal:* muscle cramps
> *Central nervous system:* tremor, headache, dizziness
> *Psychological:* hyperactivity in children, anxiety, sleep and behavioural disturbances in children
> *Blood:* low serum potassium levels
> *Skin:* nettle rash

Strength level: 2 (3 if used in severe, life-threatening attacks of asthma where there is the use of several bronchodilator medications as well as corticosteroids)

THEOPHYLLINE AND ITS RELATIVES

Theophylline is used to relieve wheezing, although there are increased side-effects when it is given together with beta-adrenoceptor stimulants (see above).

Generic name	Brand name	Dosage
aminophylline	Aminophylline, Clonofilin SR, Pecram, Phyllocontin Continus	100–300 mg 3–4 times daily
theophylline	Lasma, Nuelin, Nuelin SA, Quibron*, Quibron-T, Slo-Phyllin, Theo-Dur, Theolate*, Uniphyllin Continus, Zepholin	Depends upon the exact preparation

Table 7.4: Theophylline and its relatives

Uses: asthma

When not to be used: porphyria

Cautions: low blood pressure, heart disease, kidney disease, hyperthyroidism, stomach and duodenal ulceration, liver impairment, epilepsy, the elderly, fever

Effects
Cardiovascular: palpitations, rapid heart rate
Gastrointestinal: nausea, vomiting, poor appetite
Musculoskeletal: cramps
Central nervous system: convulsions, headache
Psychological: insomnia

Strength level: 2 (3 if used in severe, life-threatening attacks of asthma where there is the use of several bronchodilator medications as well as corticosteroids)

ANTICHOLINERGIC DRUGS (INHALED)

Anticholinergic drugs also relieve wheezing but are generally given to people who are already taking beta-adrenoceptor stimulants (see above).

Generic name	Brand name	Dosage
ipratropium bromide	Atrovent, Combivent*, Duovent*	1–2 puffs 3–4 times daily.
oxitropium	Oxivent	200 mcg 2–3 times daily

Table 7.5: Anticholinergic drugs (inhaled)

Uses: nasal conditions, asthma

Cautions: glaucoma, enlarged prostate, fever, hot weather

Effects
  Gastrointestinal: dry mouth, constipation
  Urogenital: retention of urine

Strength level: 2 (3 if used in severe, life-threatening attacks of asthma where there is the use of several bronchodilator medications as well as corticosteroids)

HOLISTIC MANAGEMENT OF ASTHMA MEDICATION

It may be difficult to make an energetic diagnosis, because the clinical picture changes so much with the medication. The emphasis should be to try to wean patients onto less powerful agents as treatment progresses. Accordingly, holistic treatment will be antidoted less and the clinical picture will become clearer.

Any corticosteroid should be withdrawn slowly, because of its powerful suppressive action and the release of symptoms that may occur when it is reduced in dosage. If the patient is taking oral forms (e.g. prednisolone), this should not be reduced by more than 1 mg each month. If the patient is taking 7 mg per day, which is quite a high dose, it may take up to a year to withdraw it. It is quite in order for people to take more of their bronchodilator (within the limitations of the maximum dose) whilst this is happening, because it will have less of a suppressant effect and will be less likely to antidote treatment. If working with the prescribing doctor, try to substitute an inhaled form for the oral whenever possible.

Next, the inhaled corticosteroid should be reduced. This should be done, if possible, by the prescription of a weaker strength inhaler. When the steroid has been stopped, you can turn to prophylactic drugs such as sodium cromoglycate (sodium cromoglicate). Reduce these slowly also, since there may well be a release of suppressed symptoms. The problems here will be less than with the steroids. If there is no suggestion of allergic disease, and some patients notice no, or very little, benefit from sodium cromoglycate (sodium cromoglicate) and the like, it can be stopped at the very beginning of drug management.

Finally, the use of the bronchodilator should be addressed. I always encourage people to use it only when necessary and after trying to deal with the wheezing situation in some other way (e.g. by rest or relaxation). There is no harm in allowing a wheeze to subside on its own. Patients can take their bronchodilator if the wheezing is severe, with other symptoms such as breathlessness.

It is imperative to be aware of the symptoms of a severe attack of asthma, as this necessitates urgent treatment. Patients may need to receive conventional drug treatment to tide them over such a crisis or receive regular treatment and monitoring by holistic practitioners. I have treated severe asthma attacks myself with acupuncture with great effect. However, people should be seen frequently and regularly (at least once daily) and closely monitored. Symptoms of concern are *breathlessness* that is:

- severe;
- acute in onset;
- progressive; and
- paroxysmal attacks occurring at night.

or if accompanied by:
- confusion;
- cyanosis; and
- a pulse rate of > 120 per minute.

CASE HISTORY

A boy aged 10 years came for treatment. He had had asthma for the previous five years. He had a cough, a runny nose, sneezing and a nasal discharge. Colds always descended onto the chest. He had had six prescriptions of antibiotics each year for the previous five years. His appetite was poor and he preferred sweet food.

Medication

Ventolin inhaler: 2 puffs four times daily
Beclazone inhaler: 2 puffs four times daily
Flixonase nasal spray: 2 sprays twice daily

Pulse: floating Lung, Kidney Yin thin
Tongue: pale body with red spots at front, white sticky coat at root to front
Diagnosis: Lung Qi Deficiency, Kidney deficiency, Damp Accumulation
Treatment principles: tonify Lung Qi, tonify Kidney, resolve Damp

Drug	Type	Uses	Strength level
Ventolin inhaler	Bronchodilator inhaler	Asthma	2
Beclazone inhaler	Corticosteroid inhaler	Asthma	3
Flixonase nasal spray	Corticosteroid nasal spray	Hay fever, persistent symptoms of runny nose, sneezing	3

The table above presents an analysis of his prescribed drugs. Here we have a common situation in the drug treatment of asthma: a combination of a bronchodilator and a corticosteroid. More severe cases may also be given oral corticosteroids. It is important to address the corticosteroids first, as these interfere with the case the most. The patient can use the bronchodilator inhaler as support during the withdrawal process.

Chinese herbal medicine

I treated the patient with Chinese herbal medicine and used a variation of Rehmannia 6 (Liu Wei Di Huang Wan) with the addition of Mai Men Dong *Tuber Ophiopogonis Japonici* and Wu Wei Zi *Fructus Schisandrae Chinensis* (Mai Wei Di Huang Wan).

Shu Di Huang *Radix Rehmanniae Glutinosae Conquitae* 24 g
Shan Yao *Radix Dioscoreae Oppositae* 12 g
Shan Zhu Yu *Fructus Corni Officinalis* 12 g
Mu Dan Pi *Cortex Moutan Radicis* 9 g
Fu Ling *Sclerotium Poriae Cocos* 9 g
Ze Xie *Rhizoma Alismatis Plantago-aquaticae* 6 g
Mai Men Dong *Tuber Ophiopogonis Japonici* 6 g
Wu Wei Zi *Fructus Schisandrae Chinensis* 3 g

Outcome

At his second visit, one month later, his chest was very good, his nose had improved, as had his appetite. At visit three, one month later, he was now down to 1 puff twice daily of the Ventolin inhaler and 1 puff twice daily of the Beclazone inhaler. He only used his Flixonase when his nose was troublesome.

At his fourth visit one month later, he had no symptoms except a tendency to eat sweet food. He continued to improve over the succeeding months. He gradually reduced his Beclazone inhaler every couple of weeks by 1 puff each time. He only took his Ventolin inhaler when he needed it for his chest symptoms. He had one flare-up of tight chest and wheezing with some phlegm when he finally stopped his Beclazone, but this settled quickly over a few days. For that time he needed to take his Ventolin inhaler twice daily. After nine months of treatment, he was well with no symptoms and needed no inhalers. He remains well some five years later.

Notes

[1] Thorax 2002; 57: 683–686.
[2] Ephedrine is a less selective stimulant of the lungs and commonly causes strong symptoms of palpitations and increased heart rate. It is no longer used commonly in the treatment of asthma.

8 CARDIAC FAILURE

Heart failure is the result of the heart being unable to pump blood efficiently and is usually due to a weakness of the heart muscle. The result is that there is less blood pumped out of the heart into the arterial system and a build-up of blood in the venous system. The main symptoms of heart failure are oedema and breathlessness.

Treatment (mildest to strongest)	Strength level
Digoxin	2
Diuretics low potency medium potency high potency	 2 2 2 or 5
Vasodilator	3
ACE inhibitor	3

Table 8.1: Drug treatment of cardiac failure

DIGOXIN

Digoxin is the only drug that strengthens the action of the heart muscle. It is derived from foxglove and herbalists still use extracts of the raw plant to treat heart failure.

Generic name	Brand name	Dosage
digoxin	Lanoxin	0.0625–0.25 mg daily

Table 8.2: Digoxin

Uses: heart failure, palpitations

When not to be used: some cases of abnormal heart rhythm

Cautions: this drug may produce abnormal heart rhythms of the type for which it was first prescribed. Low potassium levels increase sensitivity to the drug and care should be taken if diuretics, corticosteroids or carbenoxolone are prescribed at the same time.

Effects

General: apathy, tiredness, malaise, sleepiness

Cardiovascular: palpitations, rapid or slow heart rate

Gastrointestinal: poor appetite, nausea, vomiting, diarrhoea, abdominal pain, lack of blood supply to intestines causing severe abdominal pain and symptoms of shock (this is a surgical emergency)

Central nervous system: central nervous system disturbances, headache

Endocrine: breast enlargement in men

Psychological: depression, psychosis, hallucinations, confusion

Blood: low platelet count leading to bleeding into the skin, prolonged bleeding after injury and spontaneous bruising

Skin: nettle rash, scarlatiniform rash

Special senses: visual disturbances

Strength level: 2

9 EPILEPSY

There are several varieties of epilepsy that are defined by conventional medicine. The precise type is diagnosed by the clinical history and the EEG appearance.

Epilepsy is difficult to treat by means of holistic medicine, because people invariably take prescribed medication and society is very hostile to altered states of consciousness, in general, and epileptic attacks specifically. It can sometimes be of benefit if care is taken and in selected cases. All the drugs suppress symptoms such as changes in consciousness, loss of consciousness and involuntary movements and in this sense are depressant or sedating in nature. The pathology is shifted into the mental and/or emotional sphere, with effects of sedation, drowsiness, confusion, irritability or hyperactivity and deterioration of behaviour.

The danger with drug reduction is the risk of the fits returning. In about 70% of cases of epilepsy, the underlying cause has subsided, as drug withdrawal is not followed by the reappearance of fits. Unfortunately, you will not know whether your patient is one of these until after reduction. Many epileptics take a 'cocktail' of several drugs – especially in the more severe cases. The drugs may also produce epileptic attacks. This is more common with multiple prescriptions. Drugs that are stimulant in nature (e.g. antidepressants, sympathomimetic agents) may lead to a worsening of the epilepsy and therefore to larger doses of anticonvulsants than would otherwise be the case.

Type of epilepsy	Drug used	Strength level
Grand mal	carbamazepine	3
	lamotrigine	3
	phenobarbitone (phenobarbital)	3
	phenytoin	3
	primidone	3
	sodium valproate	3
Petit mal	ethosuximide	3
	sodium valproate	3
Temporal lobe	carbamazepine	3

Table 9.1: Drug treatment of epilepsy

BARBITURATES

Barbiturates are highly addictive and are rarely used nowadays. They are reserved for the treatment of severe epilepsy and to treat sleep disturbances in those who are already addicted to barbiturates.

Generic name	Brand name	Dosage
amylobarbitone (amobarbital)	Amytal, Neuramyl	100–200 mg
	Sodium Amytal	60–200 mg at bedtime
	Tuinal*	1–2 at night
butobarbitone (butobarbital)	Butibel, Butisol, Soneryl	100–200 mg at bedtime
pentobarbitone (pentobarbital)	Sopental	1–2 at night
quinalbarbitone (secobarbital)	Seconal Sodium Tuinal*	100 mg at bedtime 1–2 at night
phenobarbitone (phenobarbital)	Gardenal, Lethyl, Luminal, Solfoton	60–180 mg at night
methylphenobarbitone (methylphenobarbital)	Prominal	100–600 mg daily
primidone	Apo-Primidone, Myidone, Mysoline, Sertan	500 mg daily (maximum 1.5 g daily)

Table 9.2: Barbiturates

Uses: severe insomnia in those patients already addicted to barbiturates. Phenobarbital and methylphenobarbital are used in epilepsy.

When not to be used: insomnia (due to pain), porphyria, children, young adults, elderly and debilitated patients, patients with history of drug or alcohol abuse

Effects
General: hangover-like feelings with sleepiness, allergic reactions
Respiratory: impaired respiration and breathing
Central nervous system: dizziness, headache, loss of balance
Psychological: excitement, confusion

Strength level: 3

CARBAMAZEPINE AND ITS RELATIVES

This is a commonly prescribed drug for grand mal and temporal lobe epilepsy.

Generic name	Brand name	Dosage
carbamazepine	Carpaz, Degranol, Epimaz, Epital, Tegretol, Teri	Epilepsy: 100–1,200 mg daily Pain relief: 100–1,600 mg daily Psychiatric disorders: 400–1,600 mg daily
oxcarbazepine	Trileptal	0.6–2.4 g daily

Table 9.3: Carbamazepine and its relatives

Uses: epilepsy, neuralgia (carbamazepine)

When not to be used: those taking monoamine oxidase inhibitor antidepressants (or if these have been stopped within the previous two weeks)

Cautions: reduces the effectiveness of the oral contraceptive pill. The blood count must be checked regularly at the beginning of treatment.

Effects

General: lymphatic gland enlargement, sleepiness, fatigue, multi-organ hyper - sensitivity disorder, fever, severe allergic reaction, lethargy

Cardiovascular: palpitations, fainting, collapse, heart failure, hypertension, low blood pressure, worsening of coronary artery disease such as angina pectoris, thrombophlebitis, thrombosis, oedema, raised serum cholesterol, vasculitis (inflammation of small blood vessels that may lead to skin rashes, arthritis, bruising of the skin and kidney failure)

Respiratory: breathlessness, pneumonia

Gastrointestinal: loss of appetite, taste disturbances, nausea, vomiting, dry mouth, diarrhoea, constipation, abdominal pain, sore tongue, sore mouth, raised liver enzymes, jaundice, hepatitis, liver and spleen enlargement, weight gain, rectal irritation

Urogenital: male infertility, abnormal sperm formation, loss of libido, impotence, nephritis, kidney failure, protein in urine, blood in urine, urinary frequency, urinary retention, scanty urination, raised serum urea

Musculoskeletal: increased muscle tone, muscle weakness that can be severe and almost paralytic in nature, lupus erythematosus-like syndrome, joint pain, osteomalacia, muscle cramps

Central nervous system: dizziness, headache, tremor, speech disorders, slurred speech, peripheral neuropathy, pins and needles, aseptic meningitis (causing fever, neck stiffness and sensitivity to light), neurological abnormalities, loss of balance, spasms (especially in the face), tics

Endocrine: secretion of breast milk, breast enlargement in men, abnormal thyroid function tests (decreased thyroxine and tri-iodothyronine, increased thyroid stimulating hormone)

Psychological: hallucinations, depression, restlessness, aggression, agitation, psychosis, confusion

Blood: reduction in white blood cell count that may lead to increased infections, *increase in numbers of eosinophils (type of white blood cell)* usually denoting allergic reaction, *low platelet count* leading to bleeding into the skin, prolonged bleeding after injury and spontaneous bruising, *increase in number of white blood cells, severe acute reduction in numbers of neutrophils (type of white blood cell)* leading to severe bacterial infections that are usually fatal, *reduction in numbers of red and white blood cells and platelets* leading to anaemia, increased risk of infection and bleeding into the skin, prolonged bleeding after injury and spontaneous bruising, *lack of red blood cell production,* megaloblastic anaemia, porphyria, reticulocytosis, folic acid deficiency, *anaemia* due to destruction of red blood cells, *increase in numbers of eosinophils (type of white blood cell)* usually denoting allergic reaction

Skin: allergic skin reactions, nettle rash, exfoliative dermatitis, redness of skin, bleeding into the skin, Stevens-Johnson syndrome (fever, blistering of mouth, throat, anus and eyes), toxic epidermal necrolysis (life-threatening condition where the skin peels off in sheets leaving areas stripped of skin), sensitivity to light, erythema multiforme nodosum, changes in skin coloration, itching, acne, sweating, loss of head hair, hair growth, skin rashes

Special senses: double vision, blurred vision, rapid involuntary eye movements, cataract, conjunctivitis, tinnitus, sensitivity to noise

Strength level: 3

ETHOSUXIMIDE

Ethosuximide is sometimes used to treat petit mal epilepsy.

Generic name	Brand name	Dosage
ethosuximide	Emeside, Zarontin	500 mg daily, increasing as necessary to maximum of 2 g daily
		Children under 6 years: 250 mg daily (maximum of 1 g daily)

Table 9.4: Ethosuximide

Uses: epilepsy

Cautions: liver and kidney impairment, porphyria. Regular monitoring of blood, liver and kidney function should be performed. Patients should be told to report to their doctor if they develop fever, sore throat, mouth ulcers, bruising or bleeding.

Effects

General: apathy, drowsiness, lethargy, tiredness

Respiratory: hiccoughs

Gastrointestinal: poor appetite, gastric upset, nausea, vomiting, weight loss, diarrhoea, abdominal pain, enlargement of gums, swelling of the tongue

Urogenital: nephritic syndrome, increased libido

Musculoskeletal: systemic lupus erythematosus, stiff muscles, development of antinuclear antibodies

Central nervous system: slow movement, tremor, headache, dizziness, loss of balance

Women's health: vaginal bleeding

Psychological: depression, euphoria, irritability, hyperactivity, sleep disturbances, night terrors, inability to concentrate, aggression, paranoid psychosis

Blood: reduction in white blood cell count that may lead to increased infections, *severe acute reduction in numbers of neutrophils* (type of white blood cell) leading to severe bacterial infections that are usually fatal, *reduction in numbers of red and white blood cells and platelets* leading to anaemia, increased risk of infection and bleeding into the skin, prolonged bleeding after injury and spontaneous bruising, *increase in number of monocytes* (type of white blood cell), *increase in number of white blood cells, increase in numbers of eosinophils* (type of white blood cell) usually denoting allergic reaction

Skin: rash, Stevens-Johnson syndrome (fever, blistering of mouth, throat, anus and eyes)

Special senses: short-sightedness

Strength level: 3

PHENYTOIN

Phenytoin is used to treat grand mal epilepsy. It frequently causes side-effects and is particularly disliked because it leads to acne, hair growth, thickening of the skin of the face and swelling of the gums.

Generic name	Brand name	Dosage
phenytoin	Dilantin, Diphenylan, Epanutin, Kapseals, Pentran, Phenytex	200–500 mg daily Children: 4–8 mg/kg daily

Table 9.5: Phenytoin

Uses: epilepsy

When not to be used: liver impairment

Cautions: reduces the effectiveness of the oral contraceptive

Effects

General: fever, serum sickness, allergic reactions, sleepiness, lymph gland enlargement, lymphoma and Hodgkin's disease

Respiratory: cough, breathlessness

Gastrointestinal: nausea, vomiting, constipation, hepatitis, liver damage, raised liver enzymes, enlargement of the lips, gum enlargement

Urogenital: nephritis

Musculoskeletal: joint pains, systemic lupus erythematosus, polyarteritis nodosa, Peyronie's disease, Dupuytren's contracture

Central nervous system: slurred speech, poor co-ordination, pins and needles, vertigo, dizziness, headaches, involuntary movements, muscle spasms of neck, shoulders and trunk (leading to abnormal postures), tremor, irreversible damage to the cerebellum (causing movement disorders and loss of balance), motor twitchings, peripheral neuropathy (causing weakness and numbness), loss of balance

Psychological: confusion, nervousness, insomnia

Blood: low platelet count leading to bleeding into the skin, prolonged bleeding after injury and spontaneous bruising, *reduction in white blood cell count* that may lead to increased infections, *reduction in numbers of granulocytes* (type of white blood cell), *severe acute reduction in numbers of neutrophils* (type of white blood cell) leading to severe bacterial infections that are usually fatal, *reduction in numbers of red and white blood cells and platelets* leading to anaemia, increased risk of infection and bleeding into the skin, prolonged bleeding after injury and spontaneous bruising, macrocytosis and megaloblastic anaemia, *increase in numbers of eosinophils* (type of white blood cell) usually denoting allergic reaction, immunoglobulin abnormalities

Skin: scarlatiniform and morbilliform rashes, dermatitis, large blisters, exfoliative dermatitis, lupus erythematosus, Stevens-Johnson syndrome (fever, blistering of mouth, throat, anus and eyes), toxic epidermal necrolysis (life-threatening condition where the skin peels off in sheets leaving areas stripped of skin), coarsening of the facial features, hair growth, rash, bleeding into the skin

Special senses: rapid involuntary eye movements

Strength level: 3

SODIUM VALPROATE AND ITS RELATIVES

These drugs are used to treat all types of epilepsy and are commonly used in children.

Generic name	Brand name	Dosage
divalproex (mixture of sodium valproate and valproic acid)	Depakote	Mania: 750 mg daily Epilepsy: up to 60 mg/kg body weight per day Children aged 1–12 years: 15–45 mg/kg body weight per day
sodium valproate	Epilim, Orlept, Valpro	600 mg–2.5 g daily Children under 20 kg: 20 mg/kg Children over 20 kg: 20–30 mg/kg
valproic acid	Alti-Valproic, Convulex, Dalpro, Depakene, Depakon, Deproic, Dom-Valproic, Epival, Med-Valproic, Myproic Acid, Novo-Valproic, Nu-Valproic, Penta-Valproic	Up to 60 mg/kg body weight per day Children aged 1–12 years: 15–45 mg/kg body weight per day

Table 9.6: Sodium valproate and its relatives

Uses: epilepsy. Divalproex is also used to treat mania and to prevent migraine attacks. It is not known whether divalproex is effective or safe if used for longer than 3 weeks.

When not to be used: liver disease, family history of severe liver disease, porphyria

Cautions: kidney impairment, systemic lupus erythematosus.

Liver function tests should be performed both before treatment begins and regularly for the first six months of treatment. Serum tests for sodium valproate may need to be done, particularly in children.

These drugs are known to cause abnormalities in foetal development.

Effects

General: malaise, weakness, lethargy, sleepiness, sedation, lethargy, stupor, immune disorder

Cardiovascular: oedema, vasculitis (inflammation of small blood vessels that may lead to skin rashes, arthritis, bruising of the skin and kidney failure)

Gastrointestinal: poor appetite, increased appetite, weight increase, nausea, vomiting, gastrointestinal irritation, abdominal pain, jaundice, raised liver enzymes, pancreatitis (may be life-threatening), liver failure. The liver disturbances caused by these drugs can be fatal.

Urogenital: phosphates in the urine (cloudy urine), uric acid in the urine, sugar in urine

Musculoskeletal: systemic lupus erythematosus

Central nervous system: increased number and frequency of convulsions, tremor, convulsions, brain atrophy, loss of balance

Endocrine: Fanconi's syndrome, breast enlargement in men

Women's health: no periods

Psychological: hallucinations, aggression, confusion, hyperactivity, increase in alertness, behavioural difficulties, coma

Blood: low platelet count leading to bleeding into the skin, prolonged bleeding after injury and spontaneous bruising, *reduction in white blood cell count* that may lead to increased infections, *reduction in numbers of red and white blood cells* and platelets leading to anaemia, increased risk of infection and spontaneous bruising/bleeding, *raised serum ammonia levels, reduced clotting ability of the blood, anaemia* due to lack of red blood cell production

Skin: hair loss, exanthematous rash, toxic epidermal necrolysis (life-threatening condition where the skin peels off in sheets leaving areas stripped of skin), Stevens-Johnson syndrome (fever, blistering of mouth, throat, anus and eyes), erythema multiforme

Special senses: hearing loss

Strength level: 3

LAMOTRIGINE

Lamotrigine is used to treat grand mal epilepsy.

Generic name	Brand name	Dosage
lamotrigine	Lamictal	100–200 mg daily (maximum 500 mg daily) Children of 2–12 years: 5–15 mg/kg daily

Table 9.7: Lamotrigine

Uses: epilepsy

When not to be used: liver impairment

Cautions: kidney impairment, the elderly.

There should be regular monitoring of liver and kidney function tests and blood tests.

Effects

General: tiredness, drowsiness, allergic reactions, fever, lymphatic gland enlargement

Cardiovascular: disseminated intravascular coagulation (DIC), multiorgan failure

Respiratory: facial oedema

Gastrointestinal: nausea, raised liver enzymes, vomiting

Central nervous system: headache, dizziness, tremor, increased number and frequency of convulsions (particularly when given with other anticonvulsants), unsteadiness

Psychological: insomnia, irritability, aggression, agitation, confusion

Blood: reduction in white blood cell count that may lead to increased infections, *low platelet count* leading to bleeding into the skin, prolonged bleeding after injury and spontaneous bruising

Skin: rash, Stevens-Johnson syndrome (fever, blistering of mouth, throat, anus and eyes), toxic epidermal necrolysis (life-threatening condition where the skin peels off in sheets leaving areas stripped of skin), irreversible scarring. Patients should be closely monitored for signs of effects on the skin.

Special senses: double vision, blurred vision, conjunctivitis

Strength level: 3

VIGABATRIN

Vigabatrin is only used in combination with other anticonvulsants. It causes eye damage in over 30% of patients and also leads to severe behavioural changes.

Generic name	Brand name	Dosage
vigabatrin	Sabril	2 daily (maximum 4 g daily) Children of 10–15 kg: 0.5–1 g daily Children of 15–30 kg: 1–1.5 g daily Children of 30–50 kg: 1.5–3 g daily Children over 50 kg: 2–3 g daily

Table 9.8: Vigabatrin

Uses: epilepsy

When not to be used: visual field defects

Cautions: elderly, kidney impairment, history of psychosis, depression or behavioural difficulties.

Neurological function should be closely monitored.

Effects

General: drowsiness, fatigue

Cardiovascular: oedema

Gastrointestinal: weight gain, raised liver enzymes

Central nervous system: dizziness, headache, tremor, pins and needles, loss of balance, increased number and frequency of convulsions

Psychological: excitation, agitation, hypomania, mania, aggression, depression, abnormal thinking, paranoid reactions, poor concentration, confusion, nervousness, irritability, memory disturbance, sedation, stupor, confusion

Skin: hair loss, nettle rash

Special senses: double vision, reduced field of vision, retinal disorders, optic neuritis, optic atrophy, rapid involuntary eye movements

Strength level: 3

GABAPENTIN

Gabapentin may be used in epilepsy as a second-line drug in addition to other anticonvulsants.

Generic name	Brand name	Dosage
gabapentin	Neurontin	0.9–1.2 g daily (maximum 2.4 g daily) Children of 6–12 years weighing 26–36 kg: 900 mg daily Children of 6–12 years weighing 37–50 kg: 1.2 g daily

Table 9.9: Gabapentin

Uses: epilepsy, neurological pain

Effects

General: sleepiness, fatigue, dental abnormalities, viral infections, fever, weakness, malaise, sudden unexplained death

Cardiovascular: vasodilatation, high blood pressure, oedema

Respiratory: sore throat, coughing, pneumonia, runny nose, sneezing, facial oedema

Gastrointestinal: dry mouth, nausea, vomiting, weight increase, indigestion, poor appetite, increased appetite, sore and swollen gums, dry throat, abdominal pain, constipation, diarrhoea, flatulence, pancreatitis, raised liver enzymes

Urogenital: impotence, urinary tract infection

Musculoskeletal: muscle pain, back pain, fracture, joint pain

Central nervous system: dizziness, headache, tremor, twitching, abnormal co-ordination, vertigo, involuntary movements, increased, decreased or absent reflexes, pins and needles, double vision, loss of balance

Psychological: depression, abnormal thoughts, insomnia, mood swings, nervousness, loss of memory, confusion, anxiety, hostility

Blood: reduction in white blood cell count that may lead to increased infections

Skin: rash, abrasion, itching, acne, erythema multiforme, Stevens-Johnson syndrome (fever, blistering of mouth, throat, anus and eyes), bleeding into the skin

Special senses: rapid involuntary eye movements, amblyopia, abnormal vision

Strength level: 3

HOLISTIC MANAGEMENT OF EPILEPSY

When dealing with an individual case, do not be too intimidated by the actual label of epilepsy. It merely describes a certain group of symptoms associated with electroencephalogram (EEG) changes. EEG changes are not particularly relevant to the holistic practitioner, as they are probably very common – even in the 'normal' population. The main point is to focus on the clinical picture. Having said that, a recent EEG can be helpful as, if any abnormality has subsided, it may signify that the underlying disturbance has settled.

Once treatment is instituted and improvement begins, drug reduction may be commenced. It is helpful to use other markers of improvement when epileptic attacks are completely controlled by the drugs. These will be the general health of the person and symptoms other than 'fits'. It is essential that the patient is fully committed to dealing with the epilepsy in a holistic way and realises the need to deal with certain specific areas in order to maximise health. These include dietary changes, relaxation and resolving any relevant underlying psychological issues.

Drugs can only begin to be reduced when the patient feels ready to do so. It is important for people to make adjustments to their lifestyle, because of the risk of a recurrence of convulsions. For example, it would not be appropriate to begin drug reduction in someone who drives. Dosage reduction must be slow, to minimise the risk of an epileptic attack. It is important to involve the family, so that they are supportive in this process. Clearly, when drug withdrawal is under way the clinical situation will be less stable and the patient should endeavour to relax. They should not pursue activities that are strenuous or stressful and should generally maintain a lifestyle that is not stimulating. In this way, the risk of a 'fit' occurring is minimised.

How far it is possible to reduce dosage is dependent on each case and it is difficult to generalise. Certainly, there is improved health and fewer side-effects in cases where some measure of drug reduction is possible and, in some cases, it is even possible to lead a drug-free life. Epilepsy as a result of brain injury or after a stroke is likely to need continuing anticonvulsant treatment.

Case history[1]

A man aged 41, who was born deaf, came to be treated for headaches accompanied by nausea and a troublesome burning sensation in the pit of the stomach. The headaches had started more than 20 years before, more or less when he first began working as a dental technician. They became worse and worse until the pain was intolerable and he was suffering from daily fits.

Sometimes a throbbing head pain was the first symptom, followed by nausea, but at other times the nausea, rising from the stomach, could appear first and then turn into a heavy throbbing sensation in the head. The symptoms used to last all day if he did not take painkillers, and left him feeling stunned. He was an assertive man with a very strong personality. He made it clear that he wanted to take something as effective as, or even more effective than, the strong painkillers he was used to. He could not take time off work. Work was his religion and he had no time for anything else.

The remedy prescribed was Arsenicum Sulphuratum Flavus 30C, also called Orpiment. The dosage given was 1 pellet as soon as the symptoms appeared.

Other important and fundamental keynotes that led to the prescription included:
- restlessness;
- sleeplessness (sleeping only 4/5 hours per night);
- fastidiousness and perfectionism (others did not normally meet his standards);
- anger when contradicted;
- generation of heat;

- worry about being on time and anger if others are late;
- always on the move;
- always doing something;
- anxiety or fear of being a failure;
- longing for confidence about the future; and
- a craving for chocolate so strong that he said: 'When I eat it I'm as happy as if I've made love.'

The remedy worked well from the beginning and that is the only reason the patient managed to stay with the homoeopath. He would not have allowed any 'second try'. Threatened fits became rare and symptoms responded to an acute administration of the remedy.

Note

[1] This case history first appeared in *The Clinical Medicine Guide – A Holistic Perspective* by Dr S Gascoigne (Jigme, 2001). I am grateful to Dr Maurizio Italiano for permission to use it.

10 FEMALE SEX HORMONES

Oestrogen and progesterone[1] have been used by conventional medicine for many years. They suppress the function of the ovaries and may be used to prevent pregnancy (oral contraception). Since they suppress menstruation, they are used in the treatment of a wide range of menstrual disorders, such as painful periods, heavy menstruation, irregular menstruation and cessation of periods. They are commonly said to 'regulate the periods'. This is clearly not the case, since they prevent true menstruation.[2] Bleeding only occurs due to the withdrawal of the artificial hormone for seven days each month. The term 'withdrawal bleeding' is therefore a more accurate one.

These hormones may also be used to increase oestrogen levels around the time of the menopause, when they are normally falling. This is known as hormone replacement therapy (HRT). This is an attempt to alleviate symptoms sometimes associated with the menopause, as well as preventing or delaying the onset of osteoporosis.[3,4]

The menopause is not a disease state. It does not, therefore, have to be prevented through 'treatment' or medicalised in any way.

OESTROGENS (ESTROGENS)

Generic name	Brand name	Dosage
conjugated oestrogens (estrogens)	Premarin, Prempak-C*, Premique 5	Replacement therapy: 0.625–1.25 mg daily
ethinyloestradiol (ethinylestradiol)	Binovum, Brevinor*, Cilest, Dianette*, Eugynon 30*, Femodene*, Loestrin*, Logynon, Marviol, Mercilon, Microgynon 30*, Microlite, Minulet, Norimin*, Ovran *, Ovran 30*, Ovranette*, Ovysmen*, Premarin, Schering PC4*, Prempak-C, Tri-Minulet, Trinordial, Trinovum, Triodene	Menopausal symptoms: 10–20 mcg daily Low levels of oestrogens: 10–50 mcg daily Combined contraceptive pills: 20–50 mcg daily, depending on preparation Acne: 35 mcg daily Breast and prostate cancer: up to 3 mg daily

mestranol	Norinyl-1*	1 tablet daily for 21 days; subsequent courses repeated after 7-day tablet-free interval
oestradiol (estradiol)	Activelle*, Climara, Climagest*, Climaval, Climesse*, Cyclo-Progynova*, Dermestril, Elleste-Duet*, Elleste-Solo, Estracombi*, Estraderm MX, Estradiol Implants, Estrofem, Estrapak 50*, Evorel*, Femapak*, Fematab, Fematrix, Femoston*, Femplan-MA*, FemSeven, Kliofem*, Kliogest*, Kliovance*, Menorest, Nuvelle*, Oestradiol Implants, Oestrogel, Progynova, Sandrena, Tridestra*, Trisequens*, Zumenon	As directed
oestriol (estriol)	Hormonin*, Ovestin	As directed
tibolone	Livial	2.5 mg daily

Table 10.1: Oestrogens

Uses: contraception, hormone replacement therapy (HRT) after the menopause, acne in young females, hormone-sensitive tumours, premenstrual syndrome, infertility, habitual abortion (miscarriage), menstrual disorders, endometriosis

When not to be used: pregnancy, liver disease, severe heart or kidney disease, history of thrombosis, history of severe disturbances of liver function, jaundice or general itching during a previous pregnancy, hormone-dependent disorders, uterine or breast tumours, undiagnosed abnormal vaginal bleeding, otosclerosis

Cautions: hyperthyroidism, epilepsy, migraine, asthma, kidney and heart disease may all be affected, as fluid retention is common.

Diseases such as multiple sclerosis, epilepsy and otosclerosis may worsen during treatment. Fibroids may increase in size. Endometriosis symptoms may worsen.

Treatment must be stopped if jaundice or thrombosis develops to establish the cause.

Oestrogen used on its own (without progesterone) has a high risk of leading to uterine cancer. Use of oestrogen leads to an increased risk of breast cancer. There is a higher risk of stroke, heart attack and thrombosis in women who take oestrogen.

Breast and vaginal examination as well as blood pressure measurement should be done before this drug is prescribed. These should be repeated at regular intervals of at least every six months.

Effects
General: worsening of porphyria, severe allergic reactions, sleepiness, tiredness
Cardiovascular: oedema, thrombosis, heart attack, thrombophlebitis, high blood pressure
Respiratory: pulmonary embolism
Gastrointestinal: nausea, vomiting, abdominal cramps, bloating, jaundice, weight gain, weight loss, reduced carbohydrate tolerance, raised liver enzymes, pancreatitis, gallstones and gallbladder disease
Urogenital: changes in libido (in men: feminisation, impotence)
Musculoskeletal: leg cramps, joint pains
Central nervous system: headache, migraine, dizziness, chorea, stroke
Endocrine: breast enlargement in men
Women's health: premenstrual syndrome, vaginal thrush, vaginal discharge, breast tenderness, breast enlargement and milk production, vaginal bleeding, increase in size of fibroids, infertility, uterine cancer, breast cancer, ovarian cancer
Psychological: depression, insomnia, nervousness, irritability, mood changes
Skin: brown patches on forehead, nose and cheeks, erythema multiforme, erythema nodosum, bleeding into the skin, loss of head hair, hair growth, nettle rash, itching, rash, acne
Special senses: intolerance to contact lenses

Strength level: 2

PROGESTERONES

Generic name	Brand name	Dosage
desogestrel	Desogen, Marvelon*, Mercilon*	1 tablet daily for 21 days; subsequent courses repeated after 7-day tablet-free interval

dydrogesterone	Duphaston, Duphaston HRT, Femoston	10–30 mg daily taken at certain times during menstrual cycle
ethynodiol (etynodiol)	Femulen	1 tablet daily at same time each day
gestodene	Femodene*, Femodette*, Minulet*, Triadene*, Tri-Minulet*	1 tablet daily for 21 days; subsequent courses repeated after 7-day tablet-free interval
levonorgestrel	Eugynon 30*, Levlen, Logynon*, Microgynon 30*, Microlite*, Microval, Mirena, Neogest*, Norgeston, Nuvelle*, Ovran*, Ovranette*, Tri-Levlen, Trinordial*, Triphasil	As directed
medroxy-progesterone	Cycrin, Depo-Provera*, Femplan-MA*, Premique 5*, Provera	As directed
norethisterone	Activelle*, Binovum*, Brevinor*, Estracombi TTS*, Estrapak 50*, Evorel Conti*, Kliogest*, Micronor, Noriday, Ovysmen*, Primolut N Tablets, Trinovum*, Trisequens*, Utovlan	As directed
progesterone	Crinone, Cyclogest, Gestone, Utrogestan	As directed

Table 10.2: Progesterones

Uses: endometriosis, hormone replacement therapy, oral contraception, cancer

When not to be used: current or past history of thrombosis, cerebral vascular disease, heart attack, liver impairment, known or suspected cancer of the breast, hormone-dependent tumours, pregnancy, undiagnosed abnormal vaginal bleeding and thrombophlebitis

Cautions: breast and vaginal examination as well as blood pressure measurement should be done before this drug is prescribed. These should be repeated at regular intervals of at least every six months.

Surgery should not be performed, if possible, until at least six weeks after this drug has been discontinued.

Liver tumours have occurred in some patients, some malignant, others not.

These drugs are implicated in the enlargement of uterine fibroids, worsening or development of diabetes mellitus, increase in blood pressure, development of jaundice, lack of menstrual periods during and after treatment and appearance of depression. Epilepsy, migraine, asthma, heart and kidney disease, varicose veins, multiple sclerosis, the wearing of contact lenses and any condition that is worsened during pregnancy may be exacerbated by this medication.

Effects

General: sleepiness, severe allergic reactions
Cardiovascular: thrombophlebitis, hypertension, fluid retention
Gastrointestinal: gastrointestinal upset, nausea, weight changes, jaundice
Urogenital: thrush, changes in libido
Central nervous system: dizziness, headache
Women's health: no periods, breast discomfort, premenstrual syndrome, irregular menstruation, vaginal bleeding
Psychological: depression, insomnia
Skin: itching, acne, nettle rash, loss of head hair, brown patches on forehead, nose and cheeks, hair growth

Strength level: 2

HOLISTIC MANAGEMENT

These are powerful drugs, as are all drugs that affect the endocrine system. Although they are used to treat menstrual disorders, they frequently also cause disorders in bleeding. In my own practice, I frequently treat women who have continuous vaginal bleeding for months after being given the oral contraceptive to 'regulate' their periods.

There is considerable misunderstanding about the effects of female sex hormones and much of this is because pressure is put on patients by medical practitioners and the pharmaceutical industry. These hormones are touted as the panacea for a wide variety of disorders. In reality, the cause of many menstrual disorders is at the level of the pituitary gland or related to psychological states. Manipulating ovarian hormones is not going to treat these conditions effectively and generally leads to further and greater problems as a result.

In my opinion, no woman should be given female sex hormones without at least several checks being made. I would consider the following to be the minimum.

- There should be no contraindications to their use.
- Annual checks must be made. These will include vaginal examination, blood pressure and breast examination.
- As only about 25% of women will develop problems with osteoporosis (these tend to be those who smoke, are thin and slightly built), a process of pre-selection should be undertaken for prevention treatment.
- A full discussion of side-effects should take place before treatment is considered.
- Oestrogens must never be prescribed without progesterone, because of the greatly increased risk of cancer of the uterus. Hysterectomy obviously removes this requirement.

What can we do as holistic practitioners? We have an important role to play in education, as many women are simply not aware of the problems posed by such drugs. Pharmaceutical companies that manufacture female sex hormones too often connect themselves to well-women clinics that offer mammography, cervical smears and advice about the menopause and contraception. A neutral source of information is of benefit to women who are interested in taking control of their health.

Alternative forms of contraception can be discussed with the patient and her partner and made available.[5] In the case of HRT, holistic medicine offers effective relief of symptoms around the menopause. Education is essential, so that women are empowered to make their own decisions about their health. This must include full disclosure of the effects of female sex hormones.

The key to understanding the effects of female sex hormones is to study their energetic effects. They are cold in nature and primarily affect the pelvic and uterine area. The coldness of these drugs leads to sluggishness and stagnation of Qi and, subsequently, Blood. This explains why side-effects include thrombosis, heart attack, cancer, high blood pressure, migraine and so on. In terms of Chinese medicine, the organs they mainly affect are the Kidneys, Liver and Spleen. If patients are unable to come off these drugs, it is important to support these organs so that side-effects are minimised.

When we treat women who take female sex hormones, gradual reduction is helpful if possible and this is somewhat dependent on the formulation administered. Surgical implants last for six months or so, but there a variety of dosages that can be used.

Patches or plasters can be used less frequently and the same applies to tablets.

Problems may ensue in those women who still have a uterus. Bleeding may occur at irregular intervals as the dose is reduced, so here it necessary to stop the drug and treat as required. This is to avoid a situation where the patient experiences a lot of spotting or breakthrough bleeding whilst the dosage is reduced.

A case history involving a patient taking HRT is described on page 124.

Notes

[1] Oestrogen and progesterone, the female sex hormones are normally secreted by the ovary. There are small amounts of oestrogens also produced by the adrenal glands. They are responsible for the development of the secondary sex characteristics. Their cyclical release governs the menstrual cycle.

[2] The suppression of any discharge from the body may have serious implications for health. Homoeopathic repertories provide many remedies for the treatment of disease caused by such a suppression.

[3] The extreme focus of chemical medicine on issues such as the menopause and osteoporosis leads to increases in anxiety and fear. 'The promotion of hormone replacement therapy and oestrogen replacement therapy for osteoporosis and heart disease treatment is premature and being applied too generally. Research shows these therapies have serious risks that may outweigh the benefits, especially for low-risk women, but patients are rarely given the risk-benefit analysis and high-risk groups are not targeted' (N. Worcester et al., *Feminist Review* Summer 1992; 41: 1(26).

[4] A study suggested it might be best for women with intermediate decreases in bone density to follow an exercise and calcium regime. Exercise with oestrogen is better reserved for those with low bone density (R.L. Prince et al., *The New England Journal of Medicine* 24 October 1991; 325(17): 1189(7).

[5] The Billing's method is one of the best-known methods of natural birth control (see *www.billingsmethod.com*).

11 HAY FEVER

The drugs discussed in this section are frequently used in the treatment of hay fever (allergic rhinitis) and allergies caused by house dust, animals and so forth (perennial rhinitis). The decongestants may also be used to treat symptoms of blocked nose or sneezing of any kind. Antihistamines are used in a wide range of allergic disorders.

Treatment (mildest to strongest)	Strength level
Antihistamines	2 (1 if taken symptomatically)
Decongestants – oral	2 (1 if taken symptomatically)
Decongestants – local	2 (1 if taken symptomatically)
Anti-inflammatory drugs	2
Corticosteroids – local	3
Corticosteroids – oral (see page 51)	3

Table 11.1: Drug treatment of hay fever

ANTIHISTAMINES

These drugs block the effects of naturally occurring histamine. They are generally all sedating but the newer types have less of a sedative effect.

Generic name	Brand name	Dosage
acrivastine	Semprex	24 mg daily
astemizole	Hismanal, Pollen-eze	Not to exceed 10 mg daily
azatadine	Optimine, Zadine	1–2 mg twice daily Children 1–6 years: 250 mcg twice daily 6–12 years: 0.5–1 mg twice daily

azelastine	Astelin, Optilast, Rhinolast*	Drops: 2–4 times daily Spray: One spray into each nostril twice daily
brompheniramine	Dimotane*	4–8 mg 3–4 times daily
cetirizine	Reactine, Zirtek, Zyrtec, Zynor	5–10 mg daily
chlorpheniramine (chlorphenamine)	Aller-Chlor, Calimal, Chlortab, Chlor-Phenetron, Chlor-Contac 400*, Dristan*, Expulin*, Haymine*, Lemsip*, Novopheniram, Teldrin, Trimeton, Tripolon, Trymegen, Piriton	12–24 mg
cinnarizine	Antimet, Purazine, Stugeron	30 mg three times daily
clemastine	Aller-eze, Tavegil, Tavist	1 mg twice daily
cyclizine	Marezine, Medazine, Triazine, Valoid	50 mg three times daily
cyproheptadine	Cylert, Periactin	4 mg three or four times daily
dexchlorpheniramine	Poladex, Polaramine	2 mg 4–6 times daily
dimenhydrinate	Andrumin, Dimetabs, Dramamine, Dymenate, Gravol, Marmine, Nauseatol, Novodimenate, Travacalm, Tega-Vert, Vertab	50 mg 3–4 times daily (maximum 400 mg daily)

diphenhydramine	Allerdryl, Benadryl, Benahist, Benylin*, Betasleep, Caladryl*, Dozal, Guanor*, Histalix*, Hydramine, Hydril, Insomnal, Medinex, Nytol, Panadol Night Tablets*, Propain*, Sleep-eze, Sleepgels, Sleepia, Sominex, Teedex, Uniflu*, Unisom	Sleep disorders: 50 mg at night Other conditions: dosage varies according to preparation being used
doxylamine	Abflex-4*, Acurate*, Asic, Decapryn, Dozile, Forpyn*, Nighttime Sleep Aid, Nomopain*, Nyquil*, Sedinol*, Somnil*, Unisom, Unisom Sleep Aid, Vicks Medinite*	25–50 mg at night
fexofenadine	Allegra, Allegra-D*, Telfast	1 daily
hydroxyzine	Anxanil, Atarax, E-vista, Hydroxacen, Hyzine, Multipax, Q-hydrox, Q-Med, Quiess, Rezine, Ucerax, Vistaject, Vicerax, Vistaril	Itching: 25 mg at night, up to 25 mg 3–4 times daily Anxiety (adults only): 50–100 mg 4 times daily
levocetrizine	Xyzal	1 daily
loratadine	Clarityn, Claritin, Lorastyne	10 mg daily
mebhydrolin	Fabahistin	50–100 mg three times daily
meclizine	Antivert, Ancolan, Bonine, En-Vert, Medivert, Meclicot, Sea-legs, Vertin-32	25–50 mg when necessary. Do not repeat within 24 hours

mequitazine	Primalan	1 twice daily
methdilazine	Dilosyn, Tacaryl	8–16 mg twice daily
phenindamine	Nolahist, Thephorin	25–50 mg once to twice daily
pheniramine	Avil, Daneral, Daneral SA, Fenamine	75–150 mg daily
promethazine	Anergan, Avomine, Medised*, Night Nurse*, Pamergan P100*, Pentazine, Phenazine, Phenergan, Phensedyl Plus*, Prothazine, Sominex, Tixylix Night-time*, Q-Mazine	20–75 mg per dose
terfenadine	Aller-eze, Boots Antihistamine Tablets, Histafen, Seldane, Teldane, Terfenor, Terfex, Terfinax, Triludan	Adults: 60–120 mg daily
trimeprazine (alimemazine)	Temaril, Vallergan	10 mg 2–3 times daily (maximum 100 mg daily) Elderly: 10 mg 1–2 times daily
triprolidine	Actidil, Alleract	5–10 ml 3 times daily
tripelennamine	Pelamine, Pyribenzamine	25–50 mg 4–6 times daily. Extended release formulation: 100 mg once to twice daily

Table 11.2: Antihistamines

Uses: allergic reactions, nettle rash. They may also be used for insomnia because of their sedating effects.

When not to be used: pre-coma states, people who are taking or have recently received monoamine oxidase inhibitor antidepressants

Effects

General: sedation, lassitude, high fever
Cardiovascular: dizziness, low blood pressure, tightness of the chest, palpitations, rapid heart rate
Respiratory: thickening of mucus in chest or throat
Gastrointestinal: nausea, vomiting, diarrhoea, dry mouth, abdominal pain, indigestion, poor appetite, hepatitis, jaundice
Urogenital: urinary retention
Musculoskeletal: twitching, muscular weakness, lack of co-ordination
Central nervous system: headaches, tremor, convulsions
Psychological: depression, irritability, nightmares, excitation in children, confusion in the elderly, inability to concentrate, insomnia, anxiety
Blood: anaemia due to destruction of red blood cells, other blood dyscrasias
Skin: exfoliative dermatitis (severe skin condition characterised by fever, redness, itching and scaling of skin), sensitivity to light, skin reactions, nettle rash
Special senses: blurred vision, tinnitus

Strength level: 2

DECONGESTANTS

Generic name	Brand name	Dosage
ephedrine	CAM, Do-Do*, Dolvan*, Expulin*, Franol*, Haymine*, Secron*, Vicks Medinite*	45–180 mg daily Nasal drops: 1–2 drops into each nostril
ipratropium bromide	Atrovent, Combivent, Duovent, Rinatec	1 or 2 puffs 3–4 times daily
oxymetazoline	Dristan Nasal Mist*	Spray: 1–2 in each nostril every 8–10 hours
phenylephrine	Beechams Cold Relief Capsules*, Beechams Flu Plus Caplets*, Beechams Hot Lemon Decongestant*, Dimotapp*, Dristan Decongestant Tablets*, Isopto Frin*, Lemsip with Phenylephrine*, Minims	As directed

phenylpropanolamine	Day Nurse Capsules*, Dimotapp Elixir*, Dimotapp LA Tablets*	As directed
pseudoephedrine	Advil Cold and Flu Tablets*, Dimotane Co.*, Drixora, Galpseud, Nurofen Cold and Flu*, Robitussin Expectorant Plus*, Sudafed	As directed
xylometazoline	Otrivine-Antistin Sterile Eye Drops*	As directed

Table 11.3: Decongestants

Uses: for relief of symptoms of common colds, influenza, upper respiratory tract infections, hay fever

When not to be used: high blood pressure, severe coronary artery disease, people taking monoamine oxidase inhibitor antidepressants (or within two weeks of stopping them)

Effects
General: tiredness
Cardiovascular: increased heart rate, palpitations, chest pain due to angina
Urogenital: urinary retention, painful urination
Central nervous system: tremor
Psychological: insomnia, anxiety, sleep disturbances, psychosis, hallucinations
Skin: rash

Strength level: 2

CORTICOSTEROIDS – NASAL SPRAYS

These drugs are used in conjunction with decongestants or antihistamines. They have powerful effects and are heavily suppressive. The comments made on page 51 in relation to corticosteroid use are relevant here.

Generic name	Brand name	Dosage
beclomethasone (beclometasone)	Beclo-Rhino, Beconase, Nasobec	2 sprays twice daily
betamethasone	Betnesol	2–3 drops 3 times daily
budesonide	Rhinocort Turbohaler	2 sprays in each nostril once daily
flunisolide	Syntaris	2 sprays 2–3 times daily
fluticasone	Flixonase	2 sprays in each nostril twice daily
mometasone	Nasonex	1–2 sprays in each nostril twice daily
tramazoline	Dexa-Rhinaspray*	1 dose in each nostril 6 times daily
triamcinolone	Nasacort	2 sprays in each nostril once daily

Table 11.4: Corticosteroids – nasal sprays

Uses: hay fever, perennial rhinitis (allergy to dust, feathers, hair and so forth)

When not to be used: nasal infection, injury, after nasal surgery

Effects
Respiratory: irritation of the nose, nosebleeds, nasal ulcers, sneezing, dry nose, smell disturbances
Gastrointestinal: sore throat, taste disturbances

HOLISTIC MANAGEMENT OF HAY FEVER

Corticosteroids are the most powerful of these drugs. The effect of antihistamines and decongestants is to dry secretions. They have stronger systemic effects when taken orally. The suppression of a discharge by any method can be a powerful cause of ill health. Any drug used to suppress a discharge may, on its reduction, result in the reappearance of the discharge, often to a worse degree than originally. In addition, such suppression may well lead to the development of more severe disease. In this case, the common result is the occurrence of respiratory disease such as asthma or bronchitis. Withdrawal should be slow and any symptoms that reappear should be treated with holistic medicine. A case history of a patient taking corticosteroid nasal sprays is described on page 69.

12 HYPERTENSION

Hypertension is raised blood pressure and this is common in the Western world. Drugs are the mainstay of conventional treatment for hypertension and they are usually taken for life. Many patients cannot take their medication, however, because of side-effects. According to a survey in November 1999 sponsored by the US Association of Black Cardiologists, some 36% of patients who are treated for hypertension change medications at least once because of severe side-effects. The most commonly reported side-effects were tiredness (22%) and dizziness (21%). Dr Frank James, president of the Association of Black Cardiologists, said: 'This survey highlights the extent of the tolerability problem in hypertension, which is widespread among all patient populations, and underscores the need for the medical community to continue searching for pharmacologic alternatives. Surprisingly, the survey also presents some new challenges in treating high blood pressure, because the findings show that elevated systolic blood pressure is not being controlled to the recommended levels.' In other words, medication leads to intolerable side-effects in a significant number of patients and is often ineffective in controlling high blood pressure. However, despite this damning evidence regarding drug treatment for hypertension, Dr James still sees the need to look for further drugs.

A blood pressure reading consists of two figures (e.g. 120/80). The top figure (systolic pressure) relates to when the heart contracts, the bottom figure (diastolic pressure) to when the heart relaxes. The bottom reading is the important one, since this is the pressure that pertains to a state of relaxation. If it is high for persistent periods of time, it indicates a general heightened state of tension in the system. The systolic pressure is less important in terms of diagnosing hypertension.[1]

Conventionally, hypertension is diagnosed if the blood pressure is consistently above 160/95, although this would seem to be a low figure for someone over the age of 65 or 70.

Hypertension	Blood pressure reading
Mild	140/90 to 159/99
Moderate	160/100 to 179/110
Severe	180/110 to 209/119
Crisis	A top figure of more than 210 and/or a bottom figure of more than 120

Table 12.1: Significance of blood pressure levels

Blood pressure varies with many factors and one reading means very little. It needs to be taken over several days and allowance made for factors such as exercise or stress. Certainly, people can be monitored over six months before a final diagnosis of hypertension is made. In the UK, the British Hypertension Society recommends that drug treatment should only be initiated if the bottom figure (diastolic pressure) exceeds 100 mm during the assessment period. For pressures between 90 and 100 mm, drug treatment should only be given if there is evidence of damage to organs such as the heart or kidneys. In practice, however, people are frequently diagnosed as having high blood pressure on the basis of one reading at a level below 100 mm for diastolic pressure.

Drugs used to treat hypertension are diuretics and hypotensive agents (drugs that lower blood pressure). The precise drugs selected are frequently determined by the personal preference of the prescribing doctor. Most people attending the clinic with hypertension will be taking one or more of the drugs listed below.

There is a small group of people with so-called 'malignant' hypertension (see 'Crisis' in Table 12.1), where blood pressure levels are very high and the situation requires high doses of drugs. These cases should be treated in conjunction with medical advice, as stopping or withdrawal of the drug may lead to serious consequences.

CLONIDINE

Generic name	Brand name	Dosage
clonidine	Catapres, Catapres Perlongets Dixarit, Menograine	High blood pressure: 0.15–1.2 mg (up to 2.4 mg daily in resistant daily cases) Migraine: 100–150 mcg daily

Table 12.2: Clonidine

Uses: hypertension, migraine

Cautions: depression or a history of depression, Raynaud's disease and other disorders of the circulation (brain, heart or extremities), kidney impairment.

Clonidine must not be withdrawn suddenly, because the blood pressure may rise sharply.

Effects
> *General:* drowsiness, tiredness, fatigue
> *Cardiovascular:* fluid retention, low blood pressure, palpitations, slow pulse rate, ankle swelling, cold hands
> *Gastrointestinal:* dry mouth, constipation, nausea, vomiting, poor appetite, constipation, hepatitis
> *Urogenital:* impotence, incontinence of urine, retrograde ejaculation in men
> *Central nervous system:* dizziness, headache
> *Endocrine:* breast enlargement in men
> *Women's health:* failure of orgasm in women
> *Psychological:* euphoria, depression, restlessness at night, hallucinations, psychosis
> *Skin:* rash

Strength level: 3

METHYLDOPA

Methyldopa is an older type of hypotensive drug and has been largely superseded by newer drugs. Its main side-effect is of low blood pressure, particularly when standing. Some years ago, my mother-in-law went to the funeral of her last sibling. She was, quite naturally, emotionally upset and developed headaches. Her GP took her blood pressure and prescribed methyldopa. That evening, after one dose of the medication, she got out of bed and promptly passed out. She was unconscious for two days in hospital. Fortunately, she recovered and went on to live for many years. This story illustrates the problems that can arise from diagnosing high blood pressure too quickly, the side-effects of medication and the problems that can arise when treating the elderly.

Generic name	Brand name	Dosage
methyldopa	Aldomet, Dopamet, Meldopa, Medomet	Adults: 500 mg–3 g daily

Table 12.3: Methyldopa

Uses: hypertension, migraine

When not to be used: liver disease such as hepatitis or cirrhosis, depression

Cautions: anyone who develops fever, raised liver enzymes or jaundice should stop treatment, as fatal liver damage can occur

Effects

General: drowsiness, fever, tiredness, weakness, fever

Cardiovascular: palpitations, slow pulse rate, worsening of angina pectoris, low blood pressure (when standing), oedema, high blood pressure, inflammation of heart muscle and pericardium

Respiratory: nasal stuffiness

Gastrointestinal: nausea, vomiting, abdominal distension, constipation, diarrhoea, flatulence, colitis, dry mouth, sore or 'black' tongue, pancreatitis, enlarged salivary glands, jaundice, raised liver enzymes, hepatitis

Urogenital: decreased libido, impotence, failure of ejaculation, dark urine

Musculoskeletal: muscle pains, joint pains

Central nervous system: dizziness, fainting, headache, pins and needles, worsening of Parkinson's disease, Bell's palsy, involuntary movements, light-headedness

Endocrine: breast enlargement in men

Women's health: no periods, breast enlargement, secretion of milk from the breast

Psychological: depression, nightmares, poor concentration, psychoses, poor memory

Blood: anaemia due to destruction of red blood cells that may be fatal, *reduction in numbers of granulocytes* (type of white blood cell), *low platelet count* leading to bleeding into the skin, prolonged bleeding after injury and spontaneous bruising

Skin: rash, eczema-like rash

Strength level: 3

CALCIUM CHANNEL BLOCKERS

Generic name	Brand name	Dosage
amlodipine	Istin, Norvasc	5–10 mg daily
diltiazem	Adizem, Angiozem, Angitil SR, Britiazim, Calcicard, Cardcal, Cardizem, Coras, Diltahexal, Dilzem, Entrydil, Slozem, Tildiem, Viazem XL, Zemtard	180–480 mg daily
felodipine	Agon, Plendil, Plendil ER	5–10 mg daily

isradipine	DynaCirc, Prescal	1.25–5 mg twice daily
lacidipine	Motens	2–4 mg daily
nicardipine	Cardene	20–30 mg 3 times daily
nifedipine	Adalat, Adalat Retard, Adapine, Angiopine, Beta-Adalat*, Calcilat, Cardifen, Cardilate, Coracten, Hypolar, Nifecard, Nifensar XL, Nyefax, Nif-Ten, Procardia, Systepin, Tensipine MR, Tenif*, Vasofed	15–90 mg daily
nisoldipine	Sular, Syscor MR	10–40 mg daily
verapamil	Anpec, Berkatens, Bonceur, Calicard, Calan, Cordilox, Covera-HS, Isoptin, Q-med, Ravamil, Securon, Univer, Vasomil, Veracaps, Veralan, Verapress	120–480 mg daily

Table 12.4: Calcium channel blockers

Uses: hypertension, angina (verapamil may also be used for treatment of palpitations caused by abnormal atrial rhythms)

When not to be used: heart failure with symptoms of shock, aortic stenosis, unstable angina pectoris, during or within one month of a heart attack, acute attacks of angina, to prevent heart attacks

Cautions: heart failure, severe low blood pressure

Effects
General: lethargy, flushing, weakness, sleepiness, lymphatic gland enlargement
Cardiovascular: palpitations, rapid heart rate, slow heart rate, worsening of angina pectoris, ankle swelling, heart attack, oedema, angina, heart failure, low blood pressure, vasculitis (inflammation of small blood vessels that may lead to skin rashes, arthritis, bruising of the skin and kidney failure)
Respiratory: breathlessness, nosebleeds, stuffy nose
Gastrointestinal: nausea, altered bowel habit, jaundice, raised liver enzymes, poor appetite, constipation, diarrhoea, indigestion, vomiting, weight gain, high blood sugar, abdominal pain, gum inflammation and swelling

Urogenital: impotence, urination at night, frequent urination, sexual difficulties
Musculoskeletal: muscle pain, joint pain, muscle cramps
Central nervous system: headache, pins and needles, dizziness, tremor, difficulty walking
Endocrine: breast enlargement in men
Psychological: mood changes, poor memory, depression, hallucinations, sleeplessness, nervousness, personality changes
Blood: increase in numbers of eosinophils (type of white blood cell) usually denoting allergic reaction
Skin: rash, itching, nettle rash, sensitivity to light, severe allergic reactions, itching, reddening of the skin, erythema multiforme, bleeding into the skin, exfoliative dermatitis (severe skin condition characterised by fever, redness, itching and scaling of skin)
Special senses: visual disturbances, tinnitus, poor sight, eye irritation

Strength level: 3

BETABLOCKERS

These drugs – or beta-adrenoceptor blocking drugs, to give them their full name – interfere with receptors that are stimulated by adrenaline (epinephrine) and related substances. They, therefore, have an effect of slowing down the body, leading to tiredness, cold extremities and slow pulse. I have treated people taking betablockers who have been very severely affected, even to the point of causing confusion and dementia. They are powerful in their actions and, as they are frequently used for many years, the effect is cumulative. Their main adverse effects are on the heart, circulation, digestion and kidneys.

Generic name	Brand name	Dosage
acebutolol	Monitan, Rhotral, Sectral, Secadrex	Angina: 400–1,200 mg daily Palpitations: 400–1,200 mg daily Hypertension: 400–800 mg daily

atenolol	Beta-Adalat*, Amolin, Anselol, Antipressan, Atehexol, Atenix, Atenogen, Atenomel, Aterol, Co-tenidone*, Kalten*, Nif-Ten, Noten, Tenchlor*, Tenif*, Tenlol, Tenoret*, Tenoretic*, Tenormin, Tensig, Totamol, Totaretic*	50–100 mg daily
betaxolol	Kerlone, Korlone	20–40 mg daily
bisoprolol	Bicor, Cardicor, Emcor, Monocor, Monozide 10*, Zebeta, Ziac	10–20 mg daily
celiprolol	Celiprolol, Celectol	200–400 mg daily
labetalol	Normodyne, Presolol, Trandate	100–800 mg daily
metoprolol	Betaloc, Betazok, Co-Betaloc*, Lopressor, Minax, Toprol XL	100–300 mg daily
nadolol	Corgard, Corgaretic	Hypertension: 80–240 mg daily Angina: 40–160 mg daily Palpitations: 40–160 mg daily Migraine prevention: 40–160 mg daily
oxprenolol	Apsolox, Corbeton, Trasicor, Trasidrex*	Hypertension: 80–160 mg daily Angina: 80–160 mg daily Palpitations: 40–240 mg daily Anxiety: 40–80 mg daily

propranolol	Angilol, Apsolol, Berkolol, Beta-Prograne, Cardinol, Deralin, Detensol, Inderal, Inderal-LA, Inderetic*, Inderex*, Inderide LA, Lorol, Novopranol, Nolol, Prodorol, Pronol, Propanix, Tiperal	Palpitations: 30–160 mg daily Angina: 80–240 mg daily Hypertension: 160–320 mg daily Migraine prevention and anxiety: 80–160 mg daily
timolol	Betim, Blocadren, Cardol, Cosopt, Moducren*, Prestim*	Hypertension: 10–60 mg daily (by mouth) Angina: 10–45 mg daily Heart attack: 10–20 mg daily Migraine prevention: 10–20 mg daily

Table 12.5: Betablockers

Uses: hypertension, post-heart attack, palpitations, migraine, hyperthyroidism, glaucoma (drops). Betablockers can also be given for anxiety and phobic attacks. I have known them to be given to children for school phobia.

When not to be used: abnormal heart rhythms, history of wheezing, after prolonged fasting and in patients with diabetes mellitus. Because these drugs block the adrenaline/epinephrine response, patients cannot detect when they become hypoglycaemic – a potentially fatal situation in a diabetic who takes insulin or hypoglycaemic drugs.

Cautions: heart failure can be brought on or worsened by these drugs. The dosage should be reduced if the heart rate is slow.

They must not to be stopped suddenly if there is ischaemic heart disease. What this means, in practice, is that, where these agents have been given for a prolonged period of time (over several months), they should always be reduced slowly, because sudden withdrawal could lead to a heart attack. Since people may have ischaemic heart disease to some degree, it seems sensible to reduce slowly even in people who have been prescribed this drug for migraine or anxiety.

Effects
General: tiredness
Cardiovascular: cold hands and feet, low blood pressure, palpitations, worsening of oedema, cramping pains in feet and legs on exercise, Raynaud's phenomenon, slow

heart rate, low blood pressure that worsens with standing (sometimes leading to fainting), raised serum cholesterol levels
Respiratory: wheezing (this can be fatal in those with asthma or a history of asthma)
Gastrointestinal: diarrhoea, gastrointestinal disturbance, low blood sugar
Urogenital: impotence
Musculoskeletal: muscle weakness and fatigue (particularly after exercise), increase in ANA (antinuclear antibodies)
Central nervous system: dizziness, pins and needles in the hands
Psychological: sleep disturbances, nightmares, mood changes, confusion, hallucinations, psychoses
Blood: low platelet count leading to bleeding into the skin, prolonged bleeding after injury and spontaneous bruising
Skin: hair loss, psoriasis-like skin rash, worsening of psoriasis, bleeding into the skin
Special senses: visual disturbances, eye changes such as conjunctivitis and 'dry eye'

Strength level: 3

ANGIOTENSIN-CONVERTING ENZYME (ACE) INHIBITOR

Generic name	Brand name	Dosage
captopril	Acepril, Capoten, Acezide*, Capozide*, Aceomel, Actopril	50–150 mg daily
cilazapril	Vascace	Hypertension: 2.5–5 mg daily Heart failure: 1–2.5 mg daily
enalapril	Innovace, Innozide*, Teczem, Vasotec	10–40 mg daily
fosinopril	Staril	10–40 mg daily
lisinopril	Carace, Prinivil, Zestril, Zestoretic*	2.5–20 mg daily
moexipril	Perdix, Univasc	7.5–30 mg daily
perindopril	Coversyl	Hypertension: 2–4 mg daily
quinapril	Accupril, Accupro, Accuretic*	Hypertension: 20–40 mg daily Heart failure: 10–20 mg daily

| ramipril | Altace, Tritace, Trialix | Hypertension: 2.5–10 mg daily
Heart failure: 5–10 mg daily |
| trandolapril | Gopten, Odrik | Hypertension: 500 mcg–2 mg daily
Prevention after heart attack: 500 mcg–4 mg daily |

Table 12.6: Angiotensin-converting enzyme (ACE) inhibitor

Uses: hypertension

When not to be used: allergic oedema, autoimmune disease affecting the blood vessels, those who take immunosuppressants, kidney impairment

Cautions: all patients must have kidney function tests before treatment. This must at least include urine examination with serum urea and creatinine levels.

All patients should be specifically told to report any sign of infection, such as sore throat and fever, so that a white blood cell count can be taken.

When the drug is given to patients with previous kidney disease, monthly urinary protein estimations by 'dip stick' should be performed for the first nine months of treatment.

Effects
> *General:* serum sickness, tiredness, lymphatic gland enlargement, fever, malaise
> *Cardiovascular:* low blood pressure, palpitations, rapid heart rate, vasculitis (inflammation of small blood vessels that may lead to skin rashes, arthritis, bruising of the skin and kidney failure)
> *Respiratory:* swollen extremities, swelling of face, lips, mucous membranes, tongue, glottis or larynx, dry cough, wheezing, sinusitis, runny nose, sore throat
> *Gastrointestinal:* loss of taste, weight loss, sore mouth, mouth ulcers, raised liver enzymes, liver damage, jaundice, indigestion, abdominal pain, pancreatitis, nausea, vomiting, diarrhoea, constipation, hepatitis
> *Urogenital:* kidney impairment, protein in the urine, raised serum urea and creatinine, raised serum potassium levels
> *Musculoskeletal:* positive antinuclear antibody test, joint swelling, joint pains, muscle pains
> *Central nervous system:* dizziness, pins and needles of the hands, headache
> *Blood:* reduction of neutrophils (type of white blood cell) leading to increased susceptibility to infection, anaemia, low platelet count leading to bleeding into the

skin, prolonged bleeding after injury and spontaneous bruising, *reduction in white blood cell count* that may lead to increased infections, *anaemia* due to destruction of red blood cells, *raised erythrocyte sedimentation rate, increase in numbers of eosinophils* (type of white blood cell) usually denoting allergic reaction, increase in number of white blood cells

Skin: rash, itching, nettle rash, blistering rash (small or large), flushes, sensitivity to light

Strength level: 3

ANGIOTENSIN II RECEPTOR BLOCKERS

Generic name	Brand name	Dosage
irbesartan	Aprovel	150–300 mg daily
losartan	Cozaar	50–100 mg daily
valsartan	Diovan	80–160 mg daily

Table 12.7: Angiotensin II receptor blockers

Uses: hypertension

Effects
Cardiovascular: low blood pressure leading to fainting and light-headedness (if diuretics also used)
Respiratory: angioedema
Gastrointestinal: diarrhoea, raised liver enzymes
Urogenital: kidney impairment, kidney failure
Musculoskeletal: muscle pain
Central nervous system: dizziness, migraine
Skin: itching, nettle rash

Strength level: 3

DOXAZOSIN AND ITS RELATIVES

Generic name	Brand name	Dosage
doxazosin	Cardura	Hypertension: 1 mg (starting dose), increased gradually as necessary up to 20 mg Enlarged prostate: 1–8 mg

indoramin	Baratol, Doralese	40–100 mg daily
prazosin	Alphavase, Hypovase	High blood pressure: 0.5 mg, increased as necessary to 20 mg daily Enlarged prostate: up to 4 mg daily
terazosin	Hytrin BPH	1–10 mg daily

Table 12.8: Doxazosin and its relatives

Uses: hypertension

Cautions: kidney and liver impairment

Effects
General: fatigue, malaise, weakness, sleepiness
Cardiovascular: oedema, palpitations, chest pain, angina pectoris, heart attack
Respiratory: runny nose
Gastrointestinal: nausea, raised liver enzymes
Urogenital: urinary incontinence
Central nervous system: dizziness, headache, postural dizziness, vertigo, stroke

Strength level: 3

HYDRALAZINE

Generic name	Brand name	Dosage
hydralazine	Apresoline	Hypertension: 50–100 mg daily Heart failure: 75–300 mg daily

Table 12.9: Hydralazine

Uses: hypertension, heart failure

When not to be used: systemic lupus erythematosus and related diseases, rapid heart rate, heart failure due to mechanical obstruction or lung disease

Cautions: this drug may cause or worsen angina pectoris. Patients with coronary artery disease should only take this drug with a betablocker or similar. Use with caution in patients with coronary artery disease or cerebrovascular disease.

Prolonged treatment (i.e. more than six months) may cause a systemic lupus erythematosus-like syndrome. During long-term treatment, it is advisable to check antinuclear antibodies (blood test) and do urine analysis every six months.

The drug must be stopped in the event of skin rash, fevers and change in blood count.

This drug causes lung tumours in mice and liver and testicular tumours in rats.

Effects
General: flushing, fever, malaise, lymphatic gland enlargement
Cardiovascular: palpitations, symptoms of angina, rapid heart rate, low blood pressure, oedema, heart failure, vasculitis (inflammation of small blood vessels that may lead to skin rashes, arthritis, bruising of the skin and kidney failure)
Respiratory: blocked nose, breathlessness, pleural pain
Gastrointestinal: gastrointestinal disturbances, diarrhoea, nausea, vomiting, jaundice, enlarged liver, raised liver enzymes, hepatitis, paralytic ileus, poor appetite, loss of weight
Urogenital: proteinuria, raised serum creatinine levels, glomerulonephritis, kidney failure, retention of urine, blood in urine
Musculoskeletal: joint pain, joint swelling, muscle pain, systemic lupus erythematosus-like syndrome
Central nervous system: headache, dizziness, peripheral neuritis, polyneuritis, pins and needles
Psychological: agitation, depression, hallucinations, anxiety
Blood: anaemia, reduction in white blood cell count that may lead to increased infections, *reduction of neutrophils* (type of white blood cell) leading to increased susceptibility to infection, *low platelet count* leading to bleeding into the skin, prolonged bleeding after injury and spontaneous bruising, *anaemia* due to destruction of red blood cells, *increase in number of white blood cells, reduction in numbers of red and white blood cells and platelets* leading to anaemia, increased risk of infection and spontaneous bruising/bleeding, *enlarged spleen, severe acute reduction in numbers of neutrophils* (type of white blood cell) leading to severe bacterial infections that are usually fatal, increase in numbers of eosinophils (type of white blood cell) usually denoting allergic reaction
Skin: rash, itching, nettle rash, bleeding into the skin
Special senses: watering of the eyes, conjunctivitis, exophthalmos

Strength level: 3

MINOXIDIL

Generic name	Brand name	Dosage
minoxidil	Loniten	5 mg daily (maximum 50 mg daily)

Table 12.10: Minoxidil

Uses: severe hypertension

When not to be used: phaeochromocytoma. Minoxidil should not be used in the period immediately after a heart attack.

Cautions: can cause marked water retention leading to oedema and worsening of heart failure. It must always be given with diuretics and a restricted salt diet.

Hair growth occurs in most patients and all patients should be warned of this before treatment. Hair growth returns to normal within 1–3 months after treatment has ended.

Pericardial effusion is occasionally seen and so all patients should be periodically monitored for this.

Effects
    Cardiovascular: oedema, palpitations
    Gastrointestinal: weight gain, gastrointestinal intolerance
    Urogenital: raised serum creatinine and serum urea levels
    Women's health: breast tenderness
    Skin: rash, hair growth

Strength level: 3

DIURETICS

Diuretics remove water from the body and so mainly affect the kidneys. Potassium is lost along with the water, so potassium deficiency is not uncommon and is probably more widespread than generally realised. Potassium loss is more obvious with the more powerful drugs and potassium supplements are usually given with high-potency diuretics.

Low-potency diuretics

Generic name	Brand name	Dosage
amiloride	Amilospare, Berkamil, Midamor, Co-amilofruse*, Co-amilozide*, Burinex A*, Frumil*, Moduretic*, Buram, Moduret , Lasoride, Moducren, Navispare	5–20 mg daily
spironolactone	Aldactone, Laractone, Spiroctan, Spirolone, Spirospare, Aldactide*, Lasilactone*, Spiro-Co*	50–400 mg daily
triamterene	Dytac, Dyazide*, Dytide*, Frusene*, Kalspare*, Triam-Co*, TriamaxCo*	50–250 mg daily

Table 12.11: Low-potency diuretics

Amiloride
Uses: hypertension, heart failure, cirrhosis of the liver, nephrotic syndrome, premenstrual syndrome, glaucoma, Ménière's disease

When not to be used: those who take potassium supplements, kidney failure, severe progressive kidney disease, kidney disease due to diabetes mellitus

Cautions: kidney function tests must be carried out before treatment begins in diabetic patients.

Serum potassium levels should be checked regularly, as potassium is retained with this medication. High potassium levels lead to tiredness, confusion, muscle weakness, irregular slow pulse and, eventually, cardiac arrest.

Effects
Cardiovascular: low blood pressure when standing, raised serum potassium levels
Gastrointestinal: gastrointestinal disturbances, dry mouth
Psychological: confusion
Skin: rash

Strength level: 2 or 5, depending on the situation

Spironolactone

Uses: heart failure, liver cirrhosis, nephrotic syndrome, hypertension, ascites due to cancer

When not to be used: as amiloride (above)

Cautions: as amiloride (above)

Effects

> *General:* drowsiness, lethargy, fever
> *Gastrointestinal:* gastrointestinal intolerance
> *Urogenital:* impotence
> *Central nervous system:* headache, loss of balance
> *Endocrine:* breast enlargement in men, breast soreness, masculinisation
> *Women's health:* menstrual irregularities
> *Psychological:* mental confusion

Strength level: 2 or 5, depending on the situation

Triamterene

Uses: oedema, hypertension

When not to be used: kidney failure

Cautions: kidney and liver impairment, gout or tendency to gout, with drugs that lower blood pressure. There should be regular monitoring of serum urea, sodium and potassium levels.

Effects

> *Cardiovascular:* decrease in blood pressure, raised serum potassium levels
> *Gastrointestinal:* gastrointestinal disturbances, dry mouth
> *Urogenital:* kidney stones
> *Blood:* blood disorders
> *Skin:* rash, sensitivity to light

Strength level: 2 or 5, depending on the situation

Medium-potency diuretics

Generic name	Brand name	Dosage
bendrofluazide (bendroflumethiazide)	Aprinox, Berkozide, Neo-NaClex, Corgaretic*, Inderetic*, Inderex*, Neo-Bendromax*, Neo-NaClex-K*, Prestim*, Centyl	2.5–10 mg daily
chlorthalidone (chlortalidone)	Hygroton	Oedema: up to 50 mg daily Hypertension: 25–50 mg daily Heart failure: 25–200 mg daily
	Tenoret*	1 tablet daily
cyclopenthiazide	Navidrex, Navispare*, Trasidrex*	0.25–1.5 mg daily
hydrochlorothiazide	Accuretic, Acezide*, Capozide*, Carace, Co-Betaloc*, Co-Diovan, Cozaar Comp, Dyazide*, Esidrex, HydroSaluric, Innozide*, Moducren*, Moduretic*, Zestoretic	25–200 mg daily.
hydroflumethiazide	Aldactide*	Up to 200 mg daily
indapamide	Agelan, Natrilix, Natrilix SR	2.5 mg daily
mefruside	Baycaron*	25 mg daily
metolazone	Metenix 5	Oedema: 5–20 mg daily Hypertension: 5 mg daily
polythiazide	Nephril	1–4 mg daily
xipamide	Diurexan	20 mg daily

Table 12.12: Medium-potency diuretics

Uses: oedema, hypertension

When not to be used: low serum potassium levels, precoma associated with liver cirrhosis or Addison's disease. Not to be given to anyone taking lithium.

Cautions: caution in the elderly. Regular supervision is required with monitoring of fluid and electrolyte state to avoid excessive changes to serum potassium levels or fluid balance. In treated diabetics, a change in dosage of hypoglycaemic agents may be necessary, as these drugs raise blood sugar levels.

Effects
General: fatigue
Cardiovascular: vasculitis (severe inflammation of small blood vessels that may lead to skin rashes, arthritis, bruising of the skin and kidney failure)
Gastrointestinal: thirst, dry mouth, gastrointestinal upset, pancreatitis
Urogenital: scanty urination
Musculoskeletal: muscle pain, gout
Central nervous system: dizziness, headache
Blood: blood disorders
Skin: rash, sensitivity to light
Special senses: short-sightedness

Strength level: 2 or 5, depending on the situation

High-potency diuretics

Generic name	Brand name	Dosage
bumetanide	Burinex, Burinex K	0.5–5mg daily
co-amilofruse	Co-amilofruse	1 daily
ethacrynic acid (etacrynic acid)	Edecrin	0.5–1 mg/kg of body weight
frusemide (furosemide)	Dryptal, Froop, Lasix, Rusyde, Aridel*, Co-amilofruse*, Diumide-K Continus*, Fru-Co*, Frumil*, Lasikal*, Lasoride, Aluzine, Frumax, Frusid	20–80 mg daily or alternate days
piretanide	Trialix*	1 tablet daily
torsemide	Demedex	10–20 mg daily

Table 12.13: High-potency diuretics

Frusemide (furosemide)
Uses: hypertension, heart failure, cirrhosis of the liver, nephrotic syndrome, premenstrual syndrome, glaucoma, Ménière's disease

When not to be used: where there is no urination, severe liver disease, sensitivity to sulphonamides

Cautions: liver and kidney impairment, gout, diabetes mellitus, enlarged prostate. Potassium supplements are often needed.

Effects
General: lethargy, malaise, drowsiness, fever
Cardiovascular: low blood pressure (particularly when standing), fainting
Gastrointestinal: nausea, vomiting, gastric upset, diarrhoea, jaundice
Urogenital: excess urination, dehydration
Musculoskeletal: muscle cramps, attacks of gout, raised uric acid levels
Central nervous system: dizziness, vertigo
Endocrine: raised blood sugar
Psychological: poor concentration
Blood: severe acute reduction in numbers of neutrophils (type of white blood cell) leading to severe bacterial infections that are usually fatal, low platelet count leading to bleeding into the skin, prolonged bleeding after injury and spontaneous bruising, anaemia
Skin: rash, sensitivity to light
Special senses: tinnitus, deafness, visual disturbances

Strength level: 2 or 5, depending on the situation

HOLISTIC MANAGEMENT OF HYPERTENSION

The majority of people with hypertension can be treated holistically and are usually able to reduce or even stop their medication. Blood pressure is only one factor to be taken into account by holistic practitioners in diagnosis and treatment. It is helpful not to be over-concerned with a particular set of blood pressure readings. The overall picture is the important one. Levels of blood pressure have to be high for a long time before there is any need for concern about 'strokes' and cardiac conditions.

As usual, always wait for an improvement from the holistic treatment before the patient begins to reduce the dosage of drugs. A rebound rise in blood pressure readings may be seen whenever the dose is lessened. In some cases, the patient may also experience symptoms such as light-headedness, dizziness and headache. This is why reduction must be slow and gentle. Patients soon start to feel better, partly as a result of the treatment and partly as the drug effects lessen with the reduced dose.

Begin with the most powerful drug first. Hypotensive drugs should be dealt with initially, but do not stop them suddenly, as heart problems may occur.

Once the hypotensive drug has been stopped, move on to the diuretic. Even when the drugs are withdrawn and the patient's level of health has improved, there may still be occasional flare-ups, often resulting from stressful events at home or at work. It is not necessary for the patient to resort to drugs on these occasions. Relaxation, massage and specific treatment can all be used to help. As stated above, a short-term mildly elevated blood pressure is not going to kill people and it is possible to deal with such situations in other ways.

Regarding diuretics, it is important to determine the original condition for which they were prescribed. There is a great difference in how heart failure or simple oedema before the menstrual period are managed. The higher-potency diuretics tend to be used in more severe disease.

A reduction in diuretic dosage tends to lead to the reappearance of oedema and changes in urination patterns. It may be possible for patients to take the diuretic on a symptomatic basis for a while (e.g. every 2–3 days, as necessary). This is more likely to be possible in mild cases rather than in cases of cardiac failure. More care must be taken with severe disease, since any increase in oedema is accompanied by more severe symptoms (e.g. breathlessness, severe oedema).

I treated a man with myalgic encephalomyelitis (ME) who was prescribed Centyl for swelling in his legs. This was purely to relieve symptoms and did nothing to address any underlying disease. As he improved with acupuncture and Chinese herbal treatment, he was able to reduce the dosage of his diuretic. He took his medication on alternate days. Subsequently, he reduced the dosage to 1 tablet every 3 days. As treatment progressed, he gradually lengthened the period of time between taking tablets and, eventually, he only took a Centyl tablet when he felt he needed it.

Case history

A woman aged 66 had high blood pressure for many years and had been on medication for three years. She came for treatment because she wished to control her blood pressure with less medication. Her blood pressure was currently 180/110 on medication.

She had had her last period 11 years previously and was given female hormone replacement treatment (HRT) the year after. Her sleep was generally disturbed and she woke at 2 a.m. to pass urine. She often stayed awake for an hour or so and, as she tended to be a worrier, she could lie awake worrying about things that were on her mind.

Medication

Premarin: 2.5 mg daily
Provera: 0.325 mg daily
Atecor: 50 mg daily
Centyl: 2.5 mg daily

Pulse: Kid Yin thready, Liv floating
Tongue: generally good colour. Some red prickles at the front.
Diagnosis: Kidney Yin Deficiency, Liver Yang Rising
Treatment principles: nourish Kidney Yin, sudue Liver Yang

It is important to determine what medication people are taking and why they are taking it. An analysis of this patient's prescribed drugs follows.

Drug	Type	Uses	Strength level
Premarin	Oestrogen	Female hormone replacement therapy (HRT)	2
Provera	Progesterone	Female hormone replacement therapy (HRT)	2
Atecor	Betablocker	Hypertension	3
Centyl	Low-potency diuretic	Hypertension	2

The key to this case is the use of medication that increases blood pressure (Premarin and Provera). If these are stopped, she may find that her blood pressure will normalise or at least moderate to more normal levels. In this case, therefore, it is preferable to begin with a reduction in her HRT before moving on to the other drugs. This woman came to the first consultation clearly stating that she wanted to come off her medication. This makes the practitioner's work much easier. The situation is more difficult when a patient merely comes for relief of high blood pressure and yet does not want to reduce HRT medication.

I treated her with acupuncture and Chinese herbal medicine.

Acupuncture

LIV-3 Taichong, K-3 Taixi, Ren-4 Guanyuan, SJ-6 Zhigou, SP-3 Taibai

Chinese herbal medicine

Shu Di Huang *Radix Rehmanniae Glutinosae Conquitae* 15 g
Shan Yao *Radix Dioscoreae Oppositae* 9 g
Shan Zhu Yu *Fructus Corni Officinalis* 9 g
Gou Qi Zi *Fructus Lycii Chinensis* 9 g
Niu Xi *Radix Achyranthis Bidentatae* 6 g
Tu Si Zi *Semen Cuscutae* 9 g
Lu Jiao Shuang *Cornu Cervi Degelatinatium* 6 g
Gui Ban *Plastrum Testudinis* 9 g

At her second visit, one month later, she had loose stools, twice every morning. Her herbs had finished and she was feeling better, with an increased appetite. Her energy was good and her blood pressure was 140/90.

I changed her herbal formula slightly to:
Shu Di Huang *Radix Rehmanniae Glutinosae Conquitae* 24 g
Shan Yao *Radix Dioscoreae Oppositae* 15 g
Shan Zhu Yu *Fructus Corni Officinalis* 12 g
Mu Dan Pi *Cortex Moutan Radicis* 3 g
Fu Ling *Sclerotium Poriae Cocos* 10 g
Ze Xie *Rhizoma Alismatis Plantago-aquaticae* 3 g
Rou Gui *Cortex Cinnamomi Cassiae* 3 g

She reduced the Provera to half a daily dose.

Outcome

At visit three, one month later, her sleep had improved. She was urinating less at night and was also feeling generally calmer at night. Her blood pressure was 135/90. Her HRT medication was then reduced to:

Provera 2.5 mg daily and Premarin 0.325 mg on alternate days

At visit four, one month later, she was well. She had stopped the HRT completely the day before coming for treatment. She decided that she did not need it any more. She felt fine, with just a slight headache. She only urinated once at night now. Her energy was good and her bowels normal. Her blood pressure was 140/85.

At visit five, one month later, she was feeling very good. She would have an occasional hot flush only, with no other withdrawal symptoms from the HRT. Her mood was good. She had some dull headaches on her right temple, around the eye. These would come on when she was stressed and make her tired. Her blood pressure was 140/85. She reduced her Atecor to every second day.

On her sixth visit, two months later, she felt well. She had reduced her Atecor again because she felt so well and had now been taking no medication for the previous three weeks. She felt the best she had done for years. Her blood pressure was 160/90, which was a slight increase, but, with regular treatment and monitoring, she will be fine. This would be of more concern if her blood pressure had risen by say 20 or more points and she also had symptoms of pounding headache, red face, dizziness, red eyes or blurred vision. Her treatment continues.

Note

[1] The systolic figure is roughly 100 plus the person's age.

13 INFECTIONS

Infections are usually acute[1] illnesses frequently associated with a fever. They take many forms, depending on the area affected, the individual person, their age and their state of health. Infections are invariably treated with medications that 'attack' the organism that is deemed to be the cause.

Organism	Drugs used	Typical diseases
Bacteria	Antibacterial drug (commonly called antibiotics)	Tonsillitis, sinusitis, otitis media, bronchitis, cystitis, sexually transmitted diseases, conjunctivitis, pneumonia, meningitis, septicaemia
Fungi	Antifungal drug	Thrush, fungal infections of skin or nails (e.g. athlete's foot)
Protozoa	Antiprotozoal drug	Trichomonas infection of vagina, amoebic dysentery, giardia infection of the bowel, toxoplasmosis, pneumocystis pneumonia (PCP) affecting people with AIDS
Viruses	Antiviral drug	Cold sores (herpes simplex), genital herpes, herpes zoster (shingles), HIV infection

Table 13.1: Drugs used to treat infections

In good conventional medical practice, the precise drug used depends upon the organism responsible (or assumed to be responsible). However, it is usually the case that antibiotics are given even if bacteria are not responsible. For example, antibiotics may be prescribed in cases of the common cold, influenza, earache and so on, even if bacteria are not responsible for the condition. One in six prescriptions in the UK, for example, are for antibiotics.

The short- and long-term effects of antibiotics can be marked with a general depletion in the immune system. Subsequently, infections occur more easily and are more difficult to settle. A vicious cycle can develop where antibiotics are given for each acute flare-up leading to a recurrence some weeks or months later for which antibiotics are prescribed again.

ANTIBIOTICS

Penicillins

Generic name	Brand name	Dosage
amoxycillin (amoxicillin)	Almodan, Amix, Amoram, Amoxil, Amrit, Augmentin*, Augmentin-Duo*, Galenamox, Rimoxallin, Co-amoxiclav*, Clonomox, Oramox	Adults: 750 mg–1.5 g daily (up to 6 g daily in some short courses)
ampicillin	Ampiclox *, Ampilar, Clonamp Capsules, Magnapen*, Penbritin	0.25–1 g every 6 hours
cloxacillin	Ampliclox, Orbenin*	500 mg–1 g daily
flucloxacillin	Floxapen, Flucon, Magnapen*	250–500 mg 4 times daily
phenoxy-methylpenicillin	Calvepen	1000–2000 mg daily
pivmecillinam	Selexid	200 mg 3 times daily

Table 13.2: Penicillins

Uses: bacterial infections

Cautions: kidney impairment where the dosage may need to be reduced. Frequent use results in resistant organisms.

Effects

General: severe allergic reactions

Cardiovascular: vasculitis (inflammation of small blood vessels that may lead to skin rash, arthritis, bruising of the skin and kidney failure)

Respiratory: swelling of face and upper body

Gastrointestinal: superficial staining of teeth with syrups, nausea, vomiting, jaundice, diarrhoea, indigestion, hepatitis, diarrhoea with blood and mucus

Musculoskeletal: joint pains

Central nervous system: dizziness, headache, convulsions, pins and needles

Endocrine: nephritis

Blood: anaemia due to destruction of red blood cells, *reduction of neutrophils* (type of white blood cell) leading to increased susceptibility to infection, *low platelet count* leading to bleeding into the skin, prolonged bleeding after injury and spontaneous bruising

Skin: nettle rash (usually indicates penicillin allergy), reddened skin (if given to patients with glandular fever), skin, erythema multiforme (including Stevens–Johnson syndrome–fever, blistering of mouth, throat, anus and eyes), toxic epidermal necrolysis (life-threatening condition where the skin peels off in sheets leaving areas stripped of skin), exfoliative dermatitis

Strength level: 1 if used for short course, 2 if used long term, 5 if used for life-threatening infections

Ciprofloxacin and its relatives

Generic name	Brand name	Dosage
ciprofloxacin	Cipro, Ciproxin, Ciloxan	250–750 mg twice daily
enoxacin	Penetrex	200–400 mg twice daily
lomefloxacin	Maxaquin	400 mg daily
levofloxacin	Levaquin, Tavanic	250–500 mg 1 or 2 times daily
ofloxacin	Floxin, Ocuflox, Tarivid	200–800 mg daily
cinoxacin	Cinobac	500 mg twice daily
nalidixic acid	Mictral*, Negram, Uriben	1 g every 6 hours
norfloxacin	Noroxin, Utinor	400 mg twice daily
sparfloxacin	Zagam	200 mg daily

Table 13.3: Ciprofloxacin and its relatives

Uses: respiratory and urinary infections, sexually transmitted diseases

When not to be used: children and adolescents

Cautions: epilepsy, central nervous system disorders, history of convulsions.

May produce crystals in the urine, so patients should ensure that they drink plenty of fluids.

Effects

General: sleepiness, fever, severe allergic reactions, toxic epidermal necrolysis (life-threatening condition where the skin peels off in sheets leaving areas stripped of skin)

Cardiovascular: vasculitis (inflammation of small blood vessels that may lead to skin rash, arthritis, bruising of the skin and kidney failure), palpitations

Gastrointestinal: nausea, diarrhoea, diarrhoea with blood and mucus, vomiting, indigestion, abdominal pain, poor appetite, flatulence, difficulty swallowing, raised liver enzymes, hepatitis, jaundice, major liver disorders (including liver failure)

Urogenital: kidney impairment (such as increased serum urea or serum creatinine), kidney failure, crystals in the urine, nephritis

Musculoskeletal: joint pain, joint swelling, muscle pain, tendon inflammation causing pain, swelling and creaking on movement, tendon rupture

Central nervous system: headache, restlessness, dizziness, tremor, convulsions

Psychological: depression, hallucinations, sleep disorders, psychoses, confusion, anxiety

Blood: increase in numbers of eosinophils (type of white blood cell) usually denoting allergic reaction, *reduction in white blood cell count* that may lead to increased infections, reduction in numbers of granulocytes (type of white blood cell), *low platelet count* leading to bleeding into the skin, prolonged bleeding after injury and spontaneous bruising, *increase in number of platelets* leading to increased risk of clotting, *anaemia* due to destruction of red blood cells

Skin: rash, itching, nettle rash, sensitivity to light, erythema nodosum, erythema multiforme, Stevens-Johnson syndrome (fever, blistering of mouth, throat, anus and eyes), blisters containing blood, bleeding into skin

Special senses: visual disturbances, impaired taste and smell, tinnitus, deafness

Strength level: 1 if used for short course, 2 if used long term, 5 if used for life-threatening infections

Cephalosporins

Generic name	Brand name	Dosage
cefaclor	Distaclor	Adults: 750 mg–4 g daily
cefixime	Suprax	200–400 mg daily
cefpodoxime	Orelox	100–200 mg twice daily
cefprozil	Cefzil	500 mg daily

cephalexin (cefalexin)	Ceporex, Keflex, Kefexin	Adults: 1–4 g daily
cephradine (cefradine)	Velosef	250–500 mg 4 times daily
cefadroxil	Baxan	0.5–1 g twice daily
cefuroxime	Zinnat	250 mg twice daily

Table 13.4: Cephalosporins

Uses: bacterial infections

Cautions: marked kidney impairment

Effects

General: fever, severe allergic reactions, weakness, fainting, sleepiness, lymph gland enlargement

Cardiovascular: tightness in the chest, oedema, flushing

Respiratory: oedema of the face and upper body, breathlessness

Gastrointestinal: sore swollen tongue, heartburn, nausea, vomiting, diarrhoea, diarrhoea with blood and mucus, abdominal pain, raised liver enzymes, hepatitis, jaundice, colitis

Urogenital: nephritis, protein in the urine, raised serum urea and serum creatinine, abnormal urine analysis, itching of genitals

Musculoskeletal: joint pains

Central nervous system: headache, increased muscle tone, dizziness, pins and needles

Women's health: sore vagina with discharge, thrush

Psychological: hyperactivity, nervousness, sleep disturbances, confusion, agitation, insomnia, hallucinations

Blood: increase in numbers of eosinophils (type of white blood cell) usually denoting allergic reaction, low white cell count, *reduction of neutrophils* (type of white blood cell) leading to increased susceptibility to infection, *low platelet count* leading to bleeding into the skin, prolonged bleeding after injury and spontaneous bruising, *severe acute reduction in numbers of neutrophils* (type of white blood cell) leading to severe bacterial infections that are usually fatal, *reduction in numbers of red and white blood cells and platelets* leading to anaemia, increased risk of infection and bleeding into the skin, prolonged bleeding after injury and spontaneous bruising, *anaemia* due to destruction of red blood cells, *increase in number of lymphocytes* (type of white blood cell), *reduction in white blood cell count* that may lead to increased infections

133

Skin: nettle rash, skin rashes, itching, rash with fever and joint pains, serum sickness-like reactions, erythema multiforme, Stevens-Johnson syndrome (fever, blistering of mouth, throat, anus and eyes), toxic epidermal necrolysis (life-threatening condition where the skin peels off in sheets leaving areas stripped of skin), allergic reactions such as measles-like rash

Strength level: 1 if used for short course, 2 if used long term, 5 if used for life-threatening infections

Erythromycin and its relatives

Generic name	Brand name	Dosage
azithromycin	Zithromax	500 mg daily
clarithromycin	Biaxin Filmtab, Klaricid, Klaricid XL	500 mg daily
erythromycin	Arpimycin, Erycen, Erymax, Ery-tab, Erythrocin, Erythromid, Erythroped, Ilosone, Rommix, Stiemycin, Tiloryth, Zineryt*	1–4 g daily

Table 13.5: Erythromycin and its relatives

Uses: bacterial infections

When not to be used: marked liver impairment

Cautions: prolonged use needs regular monitoring, especially of liver function. Liver function tests should be performed in those with liver impairment.

Effects
General: severe allergic reactions
Gastrointestinal: nausea, abdominal discomfort, raised liver enzymes, jaundice, diarrhoea, diarrhoea with blood and mucus
Central nervous system: convulsions, vertigo
Psychological: hallucinations, confusion
Special senses: hearing disturbances, deafness

Strength level: 1 if used for short course, 2 if used long term, 5 if used for life-threatening infections

Sulphonamides

Generic name	Brand name	Dosage
co-trimoxazole	Bactrim, Chemotrim, Comixco, Fectrim, Laratrim, Septrin Tablets	Usually 4–6 tablets daily
sulfadiazine	Sulfadiazine	1 g daily
sulfametopyrazine	Kelfizine W	2 g once weekly

Table 13.7: Sulphonamides

Uses: urinary tract infections, middle ear infections, meningitis

Cautions: may cause severe reactions such as Stevens-Johnson syndrome (fever, blistering of mouth, throat, anus and eyes) and blood disorders

Effects

Respiratory: dry cough, shortness of breath (the drug must be stopped immediately)

Gastrointestinal: nausea, vomiting, sore mouth, hepatitis, diarrhoea, sore tongue, poor appetite, raised liver enzymes, jaundice, pancreatitis, diarrhoea with blood and mucus

Urogenital: kidney failure, crystals in the urine, kidney disorders (including nephritis)

Musculoskeletal: muscle pain, joint pain

Central nervous system: aseptic meningitis causing fever, neck stiffness and sensitivity to light, headache, convulsions, loss of balance

Psychological: depression

Blood: bone marrow depression, low platelet count leading to bleeding into the skin, prolonged bleeding after injury and spontaneous bruising, *megaloblastic anaemia, severe acute reduction in numbers of neutrophils* (type of white blood cell) leading to severe bacterial infections that are usually fatal, *reduction of neutrophils* (type of white blood cell) leading to increased susceptibility to infection, *reduction in white blood cell count* that may lead to increased infections

Skin: rash, itching, hair loss, erythema multiforme, Stevens-Johnson syndrome (fever, blistering of mouth, throat, anus and eyes), toxic epidermal necrolysis (life-threatening condition where the skin peels off in sheets leaving areas stripped of skin), sensitivity to light (the drug must be stopped immediately), bleeding into the skin. Some skin reactions have been fatal.

Special senses: tinnitus

135

Strength level: 1 if used for short course, 2 if used long term, 5 if used for life-threatening infections

Tetracyclines

Generic name	Brand name	Dosage
doxycycline	Cyclodox, Demix, Doxylar, Nordox, Ramysis, Vibramycin	100–200 mg daily
oxytetracycline	Oxytetracycline, Terramycin	250–500 mg every 6 hours
tetracycline	Achromycin, Sustamycin, Tetrabid, Tetrachel, Topicycline, Deteclo*, Mysteclin*	Infections: 1–2 g daily Acne: 250 mg–1 g daily

Table 13.8: Tetracyclines

Uses: bacterial infections

When not to be used: marked kidney impairment. It will permanently stain the teeth of children under the age of 8, therefore it should not be used in this age group for that reason.

Cautions: kidney or liver impairment, those receiving drugs that may damage the liver (oral contraceptives would be included here). Long-term treatment requires monitoring of kidney and liver function and blood. This has consequences for those who receive treatment for acne, when many months of drug therapy is given.

Effects
General: fever, severe allergic reactions
Cardiovascular: pericarditis
Respiratory: pulmonary infiltration, swelling of face and upper body
Gastrointestinal: nausea, poor appetite, vomiting, diarrhoea, raised liver enzymes, hepatitis, acute liver failure, pancreatitis, discoloration of teeth and inside mouth
Urogenital: kidney failure, nephritis
Musculoskeletal: joint pains, worsening of systemic lupus erythematosus
Central nervous system: bulging fontanelles in infants, benign intracranial hypertension, headache, light-headedness, dizziness, vertigo
Women's health: discoloration of breast milk
Blood: anaemia due to destruction of red blood cells, *low platelet count* leading to bleeding into the skin, prolonged bleeding after injury and spontaneous bruising,

reduction of neutrophils (type of white blood cell) leading to increased susceptibility to infection, *increase in numbers of eosinophils* (type of white blood cell) usually denoting allergic reaction

Skin: erythema multiforme, Stevens-Johnson syndrome (fever, blistering of mouth, throat, anus and eyes), exfoliative dermatitis (severe skin condition characterised by fever, redness, itching and scaling of skin), sensitivity to light, nettle rash, bleeding into the skin, increased pigmentation of skin and nails, discoloration of sweat

Special senses: impaired hearing, discoloration of conjunctiva and tears

Strength level: 1 if used for short course, 2 if used long term, 5 if used for life-threatening infections

Fusidic acid

Generic name	Brand name	Dosage
fusidic acid	Fucidin	500 mg three times daily

Table 13.9: Fusidic acid

Uses: bacterial infections

When not to be used: biliary tract obstruction

Cautions: liver function tests must be regularly monitored. Use with caution in patients with liver impairment or those who are also taking drugs that may affect the liver.

Effects

Gastrointestinal: gastrointestinal upsets, jaundice

Urogenital: acute kidney failure

Blood: bone marrow depression, *reduction of neutrophils* (type of white blood cell) leading to increased susceptibility to infection

Skin: rash

Strength level: 1 if used for short course, 2 if used long term, 5 if used for life-threatening infections

Trimethoprim

Generic name	Brand name	Dosage
trimethoprim	Duobact, Ipral, Monotrim, Trimogal, Trimopan, Triprimix, Bactrim*, Chemotrim*, Comox*, Fectrim*, Laratrim*, Polytrim*, Septrin*	300–400 mg daily For prevention: 100–200 mg daily

Table 13.10: Trimethoprim

Uses: bacterial infections

When not to be used: severe kidney impairment where blood levels cannot be monitored regularly, megaloblastic anaemia and other blood disorders

Cautions: impaired kidney function. Regular blood tests should be performed during long-term treatment.

Effects
General: severe allergic reaction
Gastrointestinal: nausea, vomiting, gastrointestinal upset
Blood: reduction in numbers of red and white blood cells and platelets leading to anaemia, increased risk of infection and spontaneous bruising/bleeding, *folate deficiency may be worsened, raised serum potassium levels*
Skin: itching, rash, erythema multiforme, Stevens-Johnson syndrome (fever, blistering of mouth, throat, anus and eyes), toxic epidermal necrolysis (life-threatening condition where the skin peels off in sheets leaving areas stripped of skin)

Strength level: 1 if used for short course, 2 if used long term, 5 if used for life-threatening infections

ANTIFUNGAL DRUGS

Generic name	Brand name	Dosage
amorolfine	Loceryl	Local application to nails once weekly
amphotericin (amphotericin B)	Fungilin	100–200 mg 4 times daily
fluconazole	Diflucan	50 mg daily For systemic infection: 200–400 mg once daily
griseofulvin	Grisovin	500 mg daily
itraconazole	Sporanox	100–200 mg daily
ketoconazole	Nizoral	200–400 mg daily
miconazole	Daktarin	5–10 ml 4 times daily
nystatin	Nystamont, Nystan	500,000 units 4 times daily
terbinafine	Lamisil	250 mg daily

Table 13.11: Antifungal drugs

Uses: fungal infections

When not to be used: liver disease

Cautions: liver function tests should be performed when treatment is for longer than two weeks. These should be done before treatment, after two weeks and then monthly.

Caution in the elderly and those who also take drugs that can damage the liver.

Effects
General: severe allergic reactions
Gastrointestinal: nausea
Urogenital: low sperm count
Central nervous system: dizziness, pins and needles
Endocrine: breast enlargement in men
Blood: low platelet count leading to bleeding into the skin, prolonged bleeding after injury and spontaneous bruising
Skin: exanthema, itching, loss of head hair, nettle rash, rash
Special senses: sensitivity of eyes to light

Strength level: 1 if used for short course, 2 if used regularly

METRONIDAZOLE AND ITS RELATIVES

Generic name	Brand name	Dosage
metronidazole	Anabact, Flagyl, Metrogel, Metrolyl, Metrotop, Metrozol, Rozex, Vaginyl, Zadstat, Elyzol, Nidazol	600–1,200 mg daily (by mouth) 3 g daily (as suppository)
tinidazole	Fasigyn	2g as a single dose

Table 13.12: Metronidazole and its relatives

Uses: parasitic infections (e.g. giardiasis, amoebiasis, vaginal infections)

When not to be used: diseases of the peripheral nerves

Cautions: central nervous system disease. High dose or prolonged treatment should be given only when patients can be closely monitored. There is a higher risk of peripheral nerve damage and reduction in white blood cell count that may lead to increased infections and convulsions. This drug has caused cancer in animal experiments.

Effects
    General: severe allergic reactions, drowsiness
    Respiratory: swelling of face and upper body
    Gastrointestinal: unpleasant taste in the mouth, dry mouth, furred tongue, nausea, vomiting, gastrointestinal disturbance
    Urogenital: darkening of urine
    Central nervous system: peripheral neuropathy, dizziness, headache, loss of balance, poor co-ordination
    Skin: nettle rash, rash, itching
    Blood: reduction of neutrophils (type of white blood cell) leading to increased susceptibility to infection

Strength level: 1 if used for short course, 2 if used regularly

ANTIVIRAL DRUGS

There are relatively few viral diseases that can be treated with medication. They generally have severe side-effects, as viruses live inside the cell and damage to the cell itself is inevitable. Many people with viral diseases such as tonsillitis, sore throat, common cold or influenza are prescribed antibiotics even though they are not effective.

Generic name	Brand name	Dosage
aciclovir (acyclovir)	Zovirax	1–4 g daily For prevention: 800 mg daily
famciclovir	Famvir	750–1,000 mg daily
inosine pranobex (herpes simplex only)	Imunovir	1 g 4 times daily
valaciclovir	Valtrex	1 g 3 times daily

Table 13.13:
Antiviral drugs used in herpes simplex and herpes zoster (shingles) infections

Uses: herpes simplex, varicella-zoster

When not to be used: kidney impairment, history of gout or raised uric acid levels

Cautions: it is important to drink plenty of fluids

Effects
General: fatigue, fever, drowsiness
Gastrointestinal: gastrointestinal disturbances, raised liver enzymes, nausea, vomiting, abdominal pain, diarrhoea
Urogenital: raised levels of serum uric acid, urea and creatinine, raised levels of urinary uric acid
Central nervous system: headache, neurological reactions, dizziness, tremors, convulsions, coma
Psychological: confusion, hallucinations, agitation, psychosis
Blood: decreases in blood counts
Skin: rash

Strength level: 1 if used for short course, 2 if used regularly, 5 if used for eye complications of shingles

Antiviral drugs used in HIV infection

Generic name	Brand name	Dosage
abacavir	Ziagen	300 g twice daily
didanosine	Videx	250–400 mg daily
efavirenz	Stocrin, Sustiva	600 mg daily
indinavir	Crixivan	800 mg 3 times daily
lamivudine	3TC, Combivir*, Epivir, Zeffix	1 twice daily 150 mg twice daily 100 mg daily
nelfinavir	Viracept	750 mg 3 times daily
nevirapine	Viramune	200 mg twice daily
ritonavir	Kaletra*, Norvir	600 mg twice daily
saquinavir	Fortovase Invirase	1.2 g 3 times daily 600 mg 3 times daily
stavudine	Zerit	40 mg twice daily
zalcitabine	Hivid	750 mcg 3 times daily
zidovudine	Retrovir Combivir*	500–600 mg daily 1 twice daily

Table 13.14: Antiviral drugs used in HIV infection

Abacavir

Uses: HIV infection

Cautions: liver and kidney impairment

Effects
General: allergic reactions, lethargy, fatigue, fever
Gastrointestinal: nausea, vomiting, diarrhoea, poor appetite
Central nervous system: headache

Strength level: 1 if used for short course, 2 if used regularly, 5 if used for severe cases of HIV infection

Didanosine

Uses: HIV infection

Cautions: history of pancreatitis, peripheral neuropathy causing weakness and numbness, raised levels of uric acid, kidney or liver impairment

Effects

General: weakness, allergic reactions

Gastrointestinal: pancreatitis, diarrhoea, nausea, vomiting, dry mouth, raised liver enzymes, liver failure

Musculoskeletal: raised level of serum uric acid

Central nervous system: peripheral neuropathy causing weakness and numbness, headache

Endocrine: diabetes mellitus

Special senses: damage to retina and optic nerve

Strength level: 1 if used for short course, 2 if used regularly, 5 if used for severe cases of HIV infection

Efavirenz

Uses: HIV infection

Cautions: liver impairment, severe kidney impairment, the elderly

Effects

General: sleepiness, tiredness

Cardiovascular: raised serum cholesterol

Gastrointestinal: nausea, raised liver enzymes, diarrhoea, pancreatitis

Central nervous system: dizziness, headache

Psychological: abnormal dreams, depression, psychosis, insomnia, poor concentration

Skin: rash, Stevens-Johnson syndrome (fever, blistering of mouth, throat, anus and eyes)

Strength level: 1 if used for short course, 2 if used regularly, 5 if used for severe cases of HIV infection

Indinavir

Uses: HIV infection

Cautions: liver impairment, diabetes mellitus. Plenty of fluids should be drunk to prevent kidney stones.

Effects
General: weakness, severe allergic reactions, fat loss from face, arms and legs
Gastrointestinal: nausea, vomiting, diarrhoea, abdominal discomfort, indigestion, flatulence, pancreatitis, dry mouth, taste disturbances, hepatitis
Urogenital: nephritis, kidney stones, painful urination, blood in the urine, crystals in the urine, protein in the urine
Musculoskeletal: muscle pain, inflammation of muscles, rhabdomyolysis (muscle damage characterised by pain, weakness, tenderness, contractures, fever, rapid heart rate, nausea and vomiting; may lead to kidney failure and cardiac arrest)
Central nervous system: headache, dizziness, pins and needles
Psychological: insomnia
Blood: reduction of neutrophils (type of white blood cell) leading to increased susceptibility to infection, *anaemia* due to destruction of red blood cells
Skin: rash, Stevens-Johnson syndrome (fever, blistering of mouth, throat, anus and eyes), itching, dry skin, increased skin pigmentation, loss of head hair, paronychia

Strength level: 1 if used for short course, 2 if used regularly, 5 if used for severe cases of HIV infection

Lamivudine

Uses: HIV infection

Cautions: kidney or liver impairment

Effects
General: malaise, fever
Respiratory: cough, nasal symptoms
Gastrointestinal: nausea, vomiting, diarrhoea, abdominal pain, pancreatitis, raised liver enzymes
Musculoskeletal: muscle disorders
Central nervous system: headache, peripheral neuropathy causing weakness and numbness
Psychological: insomnia

Blood: reduction of neutrophils (type of white blood cell) leading to increased susceptibility to infection, anaemia, *low platelet count* leading to bleeding into the skin, prolonged bleeding after injury and spontaneous bruising
Skin: rash, loss of head hair

Strength level: 1 if used for short course, 2 if used regularly, 5 if used for severe cases of HIV infection

Nelfinavir

Uses: HIV infection

Cautions: kidney and liver impairment, diabetes mellitus, haemophilia

Effects
General: allergic reactions, fever, fat loss from face, arms and legs
Respiratory: wheezing, facial oedema
Gastrointestinal: diarrhoea, nausea, vomiting, flatulence, abdominal pain, raised liver enzymes, hepatitis
Blood: reduction of neutrophils (type of white blood cell) leading to increased susceptibility to infection
Skin: rash, itching

Strength level: 1 if used for short course, 2 if used regularly, 5 if used for severe cases of HIV infection

Nevirapine

Uses: HIV infection

Cautions: kidney and liver impairment

Effects
General: drowsiness, fatigue, fever, severe allergic reactions
Respiratory: swelling of face and upper body
Gastrointestinal: hepatitis, jaundice, nausea, vomiting, abdominal pain, diarrhoea, raised liver enzymes
Central nervous system: headache
Skin: rash, Stevens-Johnson syndrome (fever, blistering of mouth, throat, anus and eyes), toxic epidermal necrolysis (life-threatening condition where the skin peels off in sheets leaving areas stripped of skin), nettle rash

Strength level: 1 if used for short course, 2 if used regularly, 5 if used for severe cases of HIV infection

Ritonavir

Uses: HIV infection

When not to be used: marked liver impairment

Cautions: liver impairment, diabetes mellitus

Effects
General: weakness, fever, pain, fat loss from face, arms and legs
Cardiovascular: flushing
Respiratory: sore throat, cough
Gastrointestinal: belching, nausea, vomiting, diarrhoea (can be severe), abdominal pain, taste disturbances, indigestion, poor appetite, raised liver enzymes, flatulence, dry mouth, mouth ulcers, weight loss, pancreatitis
Musculoskeletal: muscle pain, raised serum uric acid
Central nervous system: headache, dizziness, numbness and pins and needles in extremities and around mouth, increased sensitivity to touch
Endocrine: decreased levels of thyroid hormones
Psychological: sleep disturbances, anxiety
Blood: reduction in white blood cell count that may lead to increased infections, *anaemia, reduction of neutrophils* (type of white blood cell) leading to increased susceptibility to infection, *electrolyte disturbances*
Skin: rash, sweating, itching

Strength level: 1 if used for short course, 2 if used regularly, 5 if used for severe cases of HIV infection

Saquinavir

Uses: HIV infection

When not to be used: marked liver impairment

Cautions: liver impairment, diabetes mellitus

Effects
General: weakness, fever, fat loss from face, arms and legs

Gastrointestinal: diarrhoea, mouth ulcers, abdominal discomfort, nausea, vomiting, liver damage, pancreatitis, raised liver enzymes
Urogenital: kidney stones
Musculoskeletal: joint and muscle pain
Central nervous system: headache, peripheral neuropathy causing weakness and numbness, pins and needles, dizziness, seizures
Blood: low platelet count leading to bleeding into the skin, prolonged bleeding after injury and spontaneous bruising and other blood disorders, *reduction of neutrophils* (type of white blood cell) leading to increased susceptibility to infection
Skin: itching, rash and other skin eruptions, Stevens-Johnson syndrome (fever, blistering of mouth, throat, anus and eyes)

Strength level: 1 if used for short course, 2 if used regularly, 5 if used for severe cases of HIV infection

Stavudine

Uses: HIV infection

Cautions: history of peripheral neuropathy causing weakness and numbness or pancreatitis (if patient is also taking drugs that may cause pancreatitis), liver or kidney impairment

Effects
General: weakness, lymphatic gland enlargement, tumours
Cardiovascular: chest pain
Respiratory: breathlessness, influenza-like symptoms
Gastrointestinal: pancreatitis, nausea, vomiting, diarrhoea, constipation, poor appetite, abdominal discomfort, raised liver enzymes
Musculoskeletal: joint and muscle pain
Central nervous system: peripheral neuropathy, headache, dizziness
Psychological: insomnia, mood changes
Blood: reduction of neutrophils (type of white blood cell) leading to increased susceptibility to infection, *low platelet count* leading to bleeding into the skin, prolonged bleeding after injury and spontaneous bruising
Skin: rash and other allergic reactions

Strength level: 1 if used for short course, 2 if used regularly, 5 if used for severe cases of HIV infection

Zalcitabine

Uses: HIV infection

Cautions: those at risk of developing peripheral neuropathy causing weakness and numbness, pancreatitis, cardiomyopathy (enlarged heart, heart failure, palpitations, embolism), history of heart failure or liver disease

Effects
General: fatigue, fever
Cardiovascular: chest pain, palpitations, rapid heart rate, cardiomyopathy (enlarged heart, heart failure, palpitations, embolism), heart failure
Respiratory: breathlessness
Gastrointestinal: mouth ulcers, nausea, vomiting, sore throat, difficulty swallowing, poor appetite, diarrhoea, abdominal pain, constipation, dizziness, weight loss, raised liver enzymes, pancreatitis, oesophageal ulcers, rectal ulcers, jaundice, liver damage, taste disturbances
Urogenital: kidney disorders
Musculoskeletal: muscle and joint pain, raised serum uric acid
Central nervous system: peripheral neuropathy causing weakness and numbness, rigors, seizures, tremor, movement disorders, headache
Psychological: mood changes, sleep disturbances
Blood: anaemia, reduction in white blood cell count that may lead to increased infections, reduction of neutrophils (type of white blood cell) leading to increased susceptibility to infection
Skin: rash, itching, sweating, loss of head hair
Special senses: hearing and visual disturbances

Strength level: 1 if used for short course, 2 if used regularly, 5 if used for severe cases of HIV infection

Zidovudine

Uses: HIV infection

Cautions: blood toxicity (blood tests should be done at least every two weeks for the first three months of treatment and then at least monthly).

Care in vitamin B12 deficiency and kidney impairment.

Effects

General: fever, somnolence, malaise, weakness

Cardiovascular: chest pain

Respiratory: cough, breathlessness, influenza-like symptoms

Gastrointestinal: nausea, vomiting, poor appetite, abdominal pain, indigestion, diarrhoea, flatulence, liver damage, raised liver enzymes, taste disturbances, pancreatitis

Urogenital: urinary frequency

Musculoskeletal: muscle pain and weakness

Central nervous system: headache, pins and needles, neuropathy, dizziness, anxiety, convulsions

Endocrine: breast enlargement in men

Psychological: insomnia, depression, poor concentration

Blood: anaemia, reduction of neutrophils (type of white blood cell) leading to increased susceptibility to infection, *reduction in white blood cell count* that may lead to increased infections, *reduction in numbers of red and white blood cells and platelets* leading to anaemia, increased risk of infection and spontaneous bruising/bleeding, *bone marrow depression, low platelet count* leading to bleeding into the skin, prolonged bleeding after injury and spontaneous bruising

Skin: rash, pigmentation of nails, skin and inside the mouth

Strength level: 1 if used for short course, 2 if used regularly, 5 if used for severe cases of HIV infection

HOLISTIC MANAGEMENT OF INFECTIONS

The first question to ask is: what was the original conventional diagnosis? For example, penicillin is used to treat sore throats and meningitis. Antifungal agents may be used to treat 'thrush' in someone who has received previous antibiotic medications, but it may also be given to people with AIDS. The practitioner's approach will be different in each of these examples. As a general rule, there are three situations to consider: (1) acute febrile illness, (2) a previous course(s) of antibiotics for a similar or related condition and (3) regular use of antibiotics.

Acute febrile illness

If a patient has an acute febrile illness and is taking an antibiotic, the practioner can take the case and treat as usual. The vitality of the person and the severity of the original condition must be assessed. If appropriate, the patient can stop the antibiotic immediately if they are usually quite well and have a relatively mild condition. The patient can then be treated as if the case were uncomplicated.

There will be few problems of suppression to deal with and the patient can be seen every other day or whenever necessary. It may be helpful to maintain contact with the patient in the ensuing days to ensure that progress is continuing and no worrying symptoms are appearing (see page 151).

The question that arises here is that of the patient developing resistance to the antibiotic. This is the rationale behind telling patients to complete the whole course of treatment. Resistance is an issue when antibiotics are given at all and is, in fact, more likely the more often antibiotics are used and with increasing dosage. Removing the antibiotic reduces the opportunity for resistant organisms to develop. Originally, it was thought that all the bacteria had to be killed by completing the course of antibiotics. Now it is recognised that this does not happen and that bacteria develop resistance to the prescribed antibiotic extremely rapidly. Exposure to antibiotics leads to resistant organisms developing.

Over the years there have been marked changes in the length of time recommended for antibiotics to be taken. This is especially obvious with urinary tract infections. When I qualified in the mid-1970s, seven or even ten days of treatment was the rule, whereas now it is not unusual to see prescriptions of three single doses.

The main issue for practitioners is the patient, not the bacteria. The person's immune system is the key and maintaining this will ensure that the infection can be dealt with and further occurrences prevented. Stopping the antibiotics reduces the harm that they, in themselves, cause to the immune system. In addition, holistic treatment strengthens people and rectifies the underlying imbalance that led to the infection in the first place.

It is also helpful to educate people that acute illnesses can be, and are, treated by holistic medicine, that acute illnesses occurring in patients having regular treatment are often related to the chronic condition and that antibiotics may deplete a patient's energy, causing problems that will need to be dealt with at a later date.

Previous courses of antibiotics for a similar or related condition

Once the practitioner has made a diagnosis, the patient's energy should be assessed. In a patient with strong energy, the case can be reviewed after treatment. If the patient is beginning to recover by the second visit, the antibiotics can often be stopped with safety. Treatment can be continued, and the patient will need to have regular sessions of treatment after the acute episode has subsided to deal with the underlying cause of the recurrent illnesses.

In a patient with weak energy, removal of the antibiotic may cause a flare-up that cannot be adequately dealt with. In this case, the acute symptoms should be alleviated as far as possible but the antibiotic should not be interfered with. The underlying condition should be treated when the acute illness is over. In this way, the acute symptoms do not worsen because of released suppressions when the antibiotics are withdrawn.

Regular use of antibiotics

Antibiotics are given long-term for conditions such as acne, urinary tract infection and chronic lung disease. These cases can addressed as for any drug that is taken continually. Obviously, the original condition should be born in mind and regular monitoring of the infective state should be considered.

HOW TO RECOGNISE A SERIOUS SITUATION IN INFECTIONS

Table 13.15 outlines what to look for when treating a patient with an 'infection'. It is important to be more circumspect when treating children, because their symptoms can change more quickly and more frequent monitoring will be necessary. In terms of acupuncture, the practitioner would treat the person every day or so and, in the case of herbs, perhaps give enough for two or three days. The practitioner may also need to be available by telephone.

Symptoms	Comments
Fever very high	104°F (40°C) and above indicates potentially severe disease; there is strong vital energy, but the process may damage the person.
Fever mild	99–100°F (37.2–37.8°C) may indicate mild disease but could also be the beginning of severe disease in a weak person (i.e. the vital energy is too weak to generate fever).
Fever prolonged	Most fevers last a day or so. If several days elapse, then the concern is that the person is not strong enough to throw off the problem.

Dehydration	This may result from loss of fluids (e.g. diarrhoea and vomiting or lack of intake). In babies, dry skin/lips, decreased skin elasticity, strong urine, scanty urine or even dry nappy, sleepiness or lack of responsiveness should be looked for. Older people will also report thirst.
Symptom severity	The stronger the symptoms (e.g. excessive diarrhoea or vomiting), the more potentially serious they are. However, it is essential to be careful, since weak people have weak symptoms (e.g. pneumonia in the elderly or people with AIDS may present only with breathlessness and no cough or fever). Each case must be assessed carefully.
Site of symptoms	Are these in the superficial levels of the body or do they involve internal organs? If symptoms occur indicating pathology in the lung, kidney, liver, heart or central nervous system, this is clearly more worrying. In terms of Chinese medicine, it is of more concern if the symptoms occur at deeper levels of the Taiyin, Shaoyin and Jueyin.
Progression	The direction of the pathology should be assessed. Is it moving to internal organs or is it more superficial? It is of more concern if symptoms start to appear that indicate pathology at a deeper level. In the case of the respiratory system, this could manifest as a sore throat with fever progressing to a cough then breathlessness and finally confusion – an effect on the deepest level (mental).
Pulse diagnosis (Chinese medicine)	If a person with an External Pathogenic Factor and a pulse that is superficial, floating and even overflowing is treated, then after treatment the pulse would be expected to moderate. If this does not occur, it indicates that the External Pathogenic Factor may be stronger than the upright Qi. Careful assessment of the case is then necessary, as treatment is likely to be difficult. The next thing to happen may be collapse of the energy.

Table13.15: How to recognise serious conditions in acute infectious disease

Note

[1] Acute disease may be defined as a disease of rapid onset and short duration (usually with strong symptoms) that either ends in recovery or death. People who have an acute disease know that they are ill. It is clear-cut and indicates that the person is of relatively strong energy. For an acute manifestation to take place, there must be strong energy in the system. Children tend to have acute illnesses, as their energy is strong.

14 INFLAMMATORY BOWEL DISEASE

The drugs discussed in this section are used in the treatment of inflammatory bowel disease such as ulcerative colitis and Crohn's disease (known as regional ileitis in the US). Some drugs may also be used to control diarrhoea as a non-specific symptom of a bowel upset or as part of a recognised condition such as irritable bowel syndrome.

LOPERAMIDE

Generic name	Brand name	Dosage
loperamide	Arret*	Acute: 2, then 1 with each loose stool
	Imodium	4–8 mg daily in chronic cases Acute: 4 mg initially, then 2 mg with each loose stool

Table 14.1: Loperamide

Uses: diarrhoea

When not to be used: constipation, abdominal distension

Cautions: in patients with impaired liver function. May precipitate ileus and toxic megacolon in ulcerative colitis patients.

Effects
General: pain
Gastrointestinal: gastrointestinal disturbances
Skin: rash

Strength level: 2

DIPHENOXYLATE

Generic name	Brand name	Dosage
diphenoxylate	Diarphen*, Lomotil*, Tropergen*	Adults: 10 mg initially, followed by doses of 5 mg

Table 14.2: Diphenoxylate

Uses: diarrhoea

Contraindications, cautions and effects: see under morphine and its relatives (page 172)

Strength level: 1 if taken occasionally, 2 when taken regularly

SULPHASALAZINE (SULFASALAZINE) AND ITS RELATIVES

Generic name	Brand name	Dosage
mesalazine	Asacol, Pentasa, Salofalk, Asacolon	Acute: 1.5–2.5 g daily Maintenance: 750–2.4 g daily
olsalazine	Dipentum	500 mg twice daily
sulphasalazine (sulfasalazine)	Salazopyrin	500 mg 4 times daily

Table 14.3: Sulphasalazine (sulfasalazine) and its relatives

Uses: rheumatoid arthritis, ulcerative colitis, Crohn's disease (regional ileitis)

When not to be used: not to be used for infants below the age of 2

Cautions: full blood counts should be performed before treatment begins and at monthly intervals for the first three months of treatment. Liver function tests should be performed monthly for the first three months of treatment. Care in people with allergic, kidney or liver disease.

Effects
   General: fever, severe allergic reaction, lymphatic gland enlargement
   Cardiovascular: inflammation of heart muscle

Respiratory: breathlessness, cough, fibrosing alveolitis which leads to progressive breathlessness, oedema around eyes

Gastrointestinal: nausea, loss of appetite, stomatitis, parotitis, pancreatitis, hepatitis

Urogenital: crystals in the urine, blood in urine, protein in urine, low sperm count, nephrotic syndrome

Musculoskeletal: joint pains, polyarteritis nodosa, systemic lupus erythematosus

Central nervous system: headache, neuropathy, aseptic meningitis causing fever, neck stiffness and sensitivity to light, convulsions, loss of balance

Psychological: insomnia, mental depression, hallucinations

Blood: increase in numbers of eosinophils (type of white blood cell) usually denoting allergic reaction, *reduction in white blood cell count* that may lead to increased infections, *reduction of neutrophils* (type of white blood cell) leading to increased susceptibility to infection, *severe acute reduction in numbers of neutrophils* (type of white blood cell) leading to severe bacterial infections that are usually fatal, *reduction in numbers of red and white blood cells and platelets* leading to anaemia, increased risk of infection and bleeding into the skin, prolonged bleeding after injury and spontaneous bruising, *low platelet count* leading to bleeding into the skin, prolonged bleeding after injury and spontaneous bruising, *anaemia* due to destruction of red blood cells, *anaemia*

Skin: generalised skin eruptions, Stevens-Johnson syndrome (fever, blistering of mouth, throat, anus and eyes), epidermal necrolysis, itching, nettle rash, sensitivity to light, exfoliative dermatitis

Special senses: redness of the eyes

Strength level: 2

IMMUNOSUPPRESSANTS

Generic name	Brand name	Dosage
azathioprine	Azopine, Azamine, Berkaprine, Immunoprin, Imuger, Imuran	50–100 mg twice daily to a maximum of 2.5 mg/kg/day
methotrexate	Methotrexate Sodium	10–25 mg weekly

Table 14.4: Immunosuppressants

Azathioprine

Uses: organ transplantation, autoimmune diseases

Cautions: for the first two months of treatment, full blood counts, including platelets, should be done weekly or more often with high dosage or if severe kidney or liver disease is present. Later, full blood counts should be repeated each month, and certainly not longer than three-monthly.

Patients should be told to report immediately if there is any infection, bruising, bleeding or other symptoms of bone marrow depression.

Care in people with liver impairment. Regular full blood counts and liver function tests should be done.

Effects

General: general malaise, fever, shivering, increased susceptibility to infection
Cardiovascular: low blood pressure
Respiratory: inflammation of the lung (cough, breathlessness, tiredness)
Gastrointestinal: nausea, vomiting, diarrhoea (can be severe), colitis, diverticulitis, bowel perforation, pancreatitis, raised liver enzymes
Urogenital: kidney impairment
Musculoskeletal: muscle pain, joint pain
Central nervous system: dizziness, headache
Blood: bone marrow depression, reduction in white blood cell count that may lead to increased infections, *anaemia, low platelet count* leading to bleeding into the skin, prolonged bleeding after injury and spontaneous bruising
Skin: rash, hair loss

Strength level: 3 (5 if used for organ transplantation or life-threatening autoimmune disease)

Methotrexate

Uses: severe psoriasis, cancer, rheumatoid arthritis

When not to be used: severe impairment of kidney, liver (hepatitis, cirrhosis, raised liver enzymes) or blood (anaemia, low white blood cell or platelet count)

Cautions: there must be regular monitoring of full blood count, urine analysis, kidney function tests, liver function tests and methotrexate levels when high doses are given.

The drug should be stopped immediately if there is any marked fall in white blood cell or platelet counts.

Effects

    General: severe allergic reactions, fatigue, chills, drowsiness, malaise, fever, lymphatic gland enlargement, increased risk of infections, death

    Respiratory: breathlessness, dry cough, pleuritic pain, lung disease

    Gastrointestinal: mouth ulcers, nausea, abdominal distress, sore mouth, sore and bleeding gums, sore throat, diarrhoea, intestinal ulceration and bleeding, liver toxicity, raised liver enzymes, liver damage, cirrhosis

    Urogenital: loss of libido, impotence, vaginal ulcers, cystitis, blood in the urine, nephropathy, kidney failure

    Musculoskeletal: raised serum levels of urea

    Central nervous system: dizziness, headache, difficulty speaking, paralysis and weakness of muscles, convulsions, leucoencephalopathy

    Women's health: vaginitis

    Psychological: mood alteration, thought disorders

    Blood: reduction in white blood cell count that may lead to increased infections, anaemia, low platelet count leading to bleeding into the skin, prolonged bleeding after injury and spontaneous bruising, *increase in numbers of eosinophils* (type of white blood cell) usually denoting allergic reaction, *bone marrow depression*

    Skin: erythematous rashes, itching, nettle rash, sensitivity to light, skin colour changes, bleeding into the skin, telangiectasia, acne, boils, loss of head hair, herpes zoster (shingles), redness of skin

    Special senses: eye irritation, blurred vision

Strength level: 3 (5 if used for cancer treatment or life-threatening autoimmune disease)

CASE HISTORY

A man aged 46 suddenly developed rectal bleeding with loose stools. He was diagnosed with ulcerative colitis. His blood pressure was low at 80/60. His bowels would be loose for several days then he would become constipated for several days. His appetite was poor. His lower abdomen was bloated and he had a lot of flatulence of unpleasant smell.

Medication

Prednisolone: 5 mg twice daily
Asacol: 2 twice daily

Tongue: pale, slightly swollen
Pulse: empty and weak Spleen position

Diagnosis: Spleen Qi Deficiency, Damp Heat in Large Intestines
Treatment principles: tonify Spleen Qi, clear Large Intestine Damp and Heat

His prescribed drugs are analysed below.

Drug	Type	Uses	Strength level
prednisolone	corticosteroid	Inflammatory conditions	3
Asacol	sulphasalazine (sulfasalazine) relative	Ulcerative colitis, rheumatoid arthritis	2

It is important in such cases to treat first and wait for any improvement before addressing the drugs. Drug reduction that is too early and too quick, particularly of stronger drugs such as corticosteroids, will lead to a flare-up in symptoms that may be unmanageable. In addition, rapid reduction of Level 3 drugs can be harmful.

Acupuncture

I treated him with acupuncture: **ST-36** Zusanli, **SP-3** Taibai, **SP-9** Yinlingquan, **ST-25** Tianshu, **CV-12** Zhongwan.

Outcome

I discussed diet with him. As well as eating healthily, with plenty of fruit and vegetables, he was to avoid tea, coffee, alcohol, dairy products and gluten. At his second visit, two weeks later, he was eating well. He had a daily bowel movement, but there was no blood. His pulses had improved and he had more energy. His hospital consultant was reducing his corticosteroid medication and he was now on 5 mg of prednisolone daily. He was to reduce to 3 mg daily in the next month.

At his third visit, three weeks later, his bowels were fine, with no blood or mucus, and working daily. He felt well. At his fourth visit, three weeks later, he was well and had stopped his prednisolone on his hospital consultant's instructions. He had felt very tired since then, with some pressure in his lower abdomen. The most striking feature over his next few visits was the degree of tiredness that he experienced. If he did not rest during the day, he would feel really weak. This is common when corticosteroids are reduced, as they are a strong stimulant. When people take them, they feel energised, hot, with increased appetite and increased desire to be active.

After two months without the corticosteroids, his energy began to improve, his bowels were normal and he felt well. He was still taking the Asacol and the hospital consultant intended for him to continue with this for several years. However, the patient decided that he wanted to reduce it. He did so over two to three months, by one tablet at a time. He occasionally experienced a short-term episode of loose stools alternating with constipation after a dosage reduction. He never had blood or mucus in his stools. After three months, he was able to stop his Asacol and he remains well some three years later. He continues to monitor his diet and his stress levels and has gained benefit from regular meditation.

15 MIGRAINE

In terms of energetic medicine, migraine is a mixed group of conditions. There may be upper gastrointestinal symptoms such as nausea and vomiting, there may be a psychological component or an attack may be brought on by certain foods. These are treated as a single entity conventionally and similar drugs are used in most cases.

Treatment (mildest to strongest)	Strength level
Diuretic	2
Paracetamol with buclizine	2
Ergotamine	2
Tranquilliser	2
Sumatriptan	2
Methysergide	2
Clonidine	3
Betablocker	3

Table 15.1: Drug treatment of migraine

ERGOTAMINE AND ITS RELATIVES

Generic name	Brand name	Dosage
ergotamine tartrate	Cafergot*, Ergate, Ergodryl Mono, Ergomar, Ergostat, Gynergen Medihaler-ergotamine, Lingraine, Medihaler-Ergotamine, Migril*	By mouth: varies according to product, but generally 1–2 mg per dose (no more than 6 mg in 24 hours or 10 mg in 1 week) Inhaler: 6 inhalations in 24 hours or 15 in 1 week Rectally: 4 mg in 24 hours or 8 mg in 1 week

dihydro ergotamine	Dihydergot, DHE 45, Migranal (nasal spray)	Acute: 2 sprays in each nostril and again after 15 minutes if necessary (maximum 4 sprays in 24 hours and 8 in 1 week)

Table 15.2: Ergotamine and its relatives

Uses: migraine (these are used less frequently now, due to their severe effects)

When not to be used: severe arteriosclerosis, coronary artery disease, thrombophlebitis, Raynaud's syndrome, Buerger's disease, severe hypertension, hyperthyroidism, porphyria, liver or renal impairment

Cautions: should not be given regularly, except in patients with very severe attacks (which are predictable in their time of onset), as prolonged use may give rise to gangrene

Effects
General: pleural and peritoneal fibrosis
Gastrointestinal: nausea, vomiting, abdominal pain, diarrhoea
Musculoskeletal: leg cramps
Central nervous system: vertigo, headache, numbness, tingling

Strength level: 2

PIZOTIFEN

Generic name	Brand name	Dosage
pizotifen	Pizotyline, Sandomigran, Sanomigran	1.5–4.5 mg daily

Table 15.3: Pizotifen

Uses: migraine

Cautions: Glaucoma (closed-angle), predisposition to urinary retention and renal insufficiency

Effects
General: drowsiness
Gastrointestinal: increased appetite, dry mouth, nausea, constipation

Central nervous system: dizziness
Psychological: restlessness

Strength level: 2

SUMATRIPTAN AND RELATIVES

These are a powerful group of drugs with strong effects on the nervous system. I once treated a woman who took Imigran for 12 months for frequent migraine attacks. At the end of that time she began to develop signs of Parkinson's disease – stiffness, slow movement and tremor.

Generic name	Brand name	Dosage
eletriptan	Relpax	40 mg when attack occurs; repeat in 2 hours if necessary (maximum 80 mg in 24 hours)
naratriptan	Naramig	2.5 mg when attack starts; repeat in 4 hours if necessary (maximum 5 mg in 24 hours)
rizatriptan	Maxalt	10 mg when attack starts; repeat in 2 hours if necessary (maximum 20 mg in 24 hours)
sumatriptan	Imigran, Imitrex	100 mg per attack (repeat if another attack occurs, up to a maximum of 300 mg in 24 hours)
zolmitriptan	Zomig	2.5 mg when attack starts; repeat in 2 hours if necessary (maximum 5 mg in 24 hours)

Table 15.4: Sumatriptan and its relatives

Uses: migraine

When not to be used: previous stroke or transient ischaemic attack, peripheral vascular disease

Cautions: kidney impairment, sensitivity to sulphonamide antibiotics, not within 24 hours of taking ergotamine

Effects
General: pain, pressure, tightness, flushing and feelings of heat, weakness, fatigue, drowsiness
Cardiovascular: increases in blood pressure
Gastrointestinal: nausea, vomiting, raised liver enzymes

Central nervous system: tingling, dizziness, pins and needles, convulsions

Strength level: 2

METHYSERGIDE

Generic name	Brand name	Dosage
methysergide	Deseril, Sansert	1–2 mg 3 times daily

Table 15.5: Methysergide

Uses: migraine (under hospital supervision only)

When not to be used: kidney, liver, lung, heart and circulatory cardiovascular disease, severe high blood pressure, autoimmune disease, cellulitis, urinary disorders, low body weight, infection

Cautions: history of stomach and duodenal ulceration. Do not stop suddenly. After six months of treatment, reduce gradually over two to three weeks to reassess the case. Do not restart for at least a month.

Effects
    General: drowsiness
    Cardiovascular: oedema, arterial spasm, angina, heart attack, low blood pressure (particularly on standing), palpitations, rapid heart rate
    Gastrointestinal: heartburn, nausea, vomiting, abdominal discomfort, weight gain, retroperitoneal fibrosis
    Musculoskeletal: cramps
    Central nervous system: dizziness, pins and needles
    Psychological: thought disorders, disturbed behaviour, insomnia
    Skin: rash, loss of head hair

Strength level: 2

HOLISTIC MANAGEMENT

Holistic treatment is generally simpler when drugs are taken symptomatically for the onset of a migraine headache. Here the situation can be dealt with as if it were a simple pain reliever. The case should be taken as usual, treated appropriately and the drugs will be used less often as the patient begins to improve. It is helpful to suggest other ways of dealing with migraine, particularly in the case of powerful drugs such as sumatriptan and its relatives. Rest, relaxation, massage and so forth can remove the need for drugs in some cases.

Treatment is more difficult where patients take drugs regularly to prevent the onset of headaches and migraine. In such cases, it may be necessary to reduce the dosage slightly until symptoms appear in order to make an accurate diagnosis.

CASE HISTORY

A man aged 42 came for treatment complaining of severe migraine headaches for the previous five years. They started over the right eye or over both eyes and could last anything up to two weeks. The longest period of time he had been pain-free was 21 days. The headaches were very severe and he had great sensitivity to noise and light when they occurred. He would vomit with them. They were very sharp and throbbing in nature. He had to lie completely still with them. They had begun after a road traffic accident some 12 years previously. His neck was constantly painful and, during a headache, was stiff and extremely tender. His bowels were constantly constipated and could miss two or three days. His energy was low. Even when there was no severe headache, there was a constant dull ache in his head.

Medication

Voltarol: one twice daily
Paracetamol: 2 four times daily
Sanomigran: 1 three times daily
Xanax: 0.25 mg three times daily
Largactil: 100 mg twice daily
Pethidine injections during an attack

Pulse: thready, especially on the right
Tongue: pale, flabby, reddish centre
Diagnosis: Qi Xu, Liver Qi Stagnation, Blood Stagnation
Treatment principles: tonify Qi, move Liver Qi, move Blood

It is important to determine what medication people are taking and why they are taking it. An analysis of this patient's prescribed drugs follows.

Drug	Type	Uses	Strength level
Voltarol	Non-steroidal anti-inflammatory drug	Pain relief (mild to moderate)	2
paracetamol	Pain reliever	Pain relief (mild to moderate)	2
Sanomigran	Migraine prevention	Migraine	2
Xanax	'Minor' tranquilliser	Anxiety	2
Largactil	'Major' tranquilliser	Sedation, schizophrenia	2 here but 4 if used in psychotic illness
pethidine	opiate	Pain relief (mild to moderate)	2

The main consideration here is the number and strength of the patient's medications. He is taking a 'minor' tranquilliser (Xanax) that is used to treat anxiety, a 'major' tranquilliser (Largactil), two pain relievers (paracetamol and Voltarol – a non-steroidal anti-inflammatory drug) and a specific drug to prevent migraine attacks (Sanomigran). Despite this heavy medication, he is still having migraines for up to two weeks every three weeks or less. In such cases, it is common that the medication itself causes headaches. The use of pethidine, which is highly addictive, is only complicating the situation further. The use of tranquillisers in painful conditions notoriously leads to depression and is not generally helpful. It is important to find out the reason why Largactil is prescribed, as it is used in schizophrenia. In this case, it is difficult to see the rationale for its use.

Acupuncture and Chinese herbal medicine

I treated him with acupuncture and with Chinese herbal medicine.

Acupuncture treatment: **G.B.-20R** Fengchi, **G.B.-21** Jianjing, **DU-14** Dazhui, **UB-18** Ganshu, **UB-17** Geshu, **UB-20** Pishu.

At his second visit, two weeks later, he felt less pressure generally in his head but there had been a severe headache that lasted three days. At visit three, two weeks later, he was fine for seven days after treatment and felt better than he had for a long time. His mood was better and he was able to do more. He had a recurrence of the headache 10 days after treatment. At visit four, two weeks later, he had felt nauseous and tired after his acupuncture treatment. He had had a sore head for several days between treatments. I gave him a Chinese herbal formula: Xiao Yao Wan plus Chen Xiang.

At his fifth visit, his bowels were much improved. He still felt tired, but his stomach was fine. His neck was very tight and sore. At the sixth visit, two weeks later, he said that he felt great, with good energy. He had some sensitivity in the head now and again but no severe pain.

At visit seven, four weeks later, he had had only one headache since the previous treatment. This had lasted one day. In between, he had been fine. Generally, the headaches were much less frequent, less severe and of a shorter duration. He was finding that he needed fewer pain relievers and he was not receiving any pethidine for the headaches. He was still taking his regular medication of Xanax, Largactil, Sanomigran and Voltarol.

At visit eight, four weeks later, he had had a miserable few weeks with pain behind his right eye. He had needed injections for headaches that had lasted three days. At visit nine, four weeks later, he felt very well. He had had no attack of pain, his neck was much more relaxed, with no stiffness or pain. He was energetic and active.

At his tenth visit, one month later, he felt very well. He had decided to stop his tablets and had thrown them away. He had had occasional headaches, lasting only two hours, and had not needed strong pain relievers. He found that an occasional paracetamol controlled the pain. His energy was good.

At his twelfth visit, two months later, he felt fine. He was able to do much more. He had had only one headache in that time, which had lasted for two hours. It had been quite painful but had settled.

Outcome

His treatment continues. Here we have a situation where the treatment is helping his condition and his pain is less. Therefore, he was able to take reduced dosages of pain relievers. However, it is frequently the case that only when the patient reaches a certain level of health will they then take charge of the situation. Here, the patient stopped all his medication and he was fine because of the treatment he had already received. Technically, it may have been better to reduce the medication slowly, in turn, but often events are overtaken when the patient takes control. It is therefore essential that you know which drugs can be stopped suddenly with no threat to life and those that cannot. The classification of drug strengths on pages 19–23 gives this information. The worst thing that can happen in a case such as this is that the migraines become more frequent or more painful.

16 PAIN RELIEF

Pain relievers are widely available and are used in the treatment of pain. Aspirin and paracetamol are also used to relieve fever. Many formulations that contain these drugs are available over the counter (for example, there are over 100 medications available that contain aspirin). When taken occasionally for the relief of pain, there will be minimal harmful effects, but they are often used regularly, daily and in significant doses.

ASPIRIN

Generic name	Brand name	Dosage
aspirin	Angettes, Caprin, Disprin, Nu-Seals, Anadin, Aspav, Codis, Equagesic, Veganin, Ascriptin, Aspro, Cox Dispersible Aspirin, Dristan, Resprin (suppositories)	Relief of pain or fever: 300–900 mg per dose Prevention of blood clots: 75–300 mg daily

Table 16.1: Aspirin

Uses: mild to moderate pain, fever

When not to be used: stomach or duodenal ulcer, haemophilia, kidney impairment in children under the age of 12 because of the risk of Reye's syndrome. This is a potentially fatal condition leading to liver and kidney damage. Reye's syndrome is mainly seen in children between the ages of 6 months and 15 years.

Cautions: history of peptic ulceration

Effects
General: allergic reactions, lymphatic gland enlargement
Cardiovascular: low blood pressure
Respiratory: wheezing, breathlessness, nasal polyps
Gastrointestinal: nausea, vomiting, indigestion, vomiting blood (this can be fatal), diarrhoea, bleeding from bowel
Central nervous system: dizziness
Skin: rash
Special senses: tinnitus

Strength level: 2 (1 if taken symptomatically)

MORPHINE AND ITS RELATIVES

Generic name	Brand name	Dosage
co-codamol* (mixture of codeine and paracetamol)	Kapake*, Solpadol*, Tylex*	1–2 every 4 hours to a maximum of 8 daily
co-codaprin* (mixture of codeine and aspirin)	–	1–2 every 4 hours to a maximum of 8 daily
codeine	Benylin with Codeine*, Co-codamol*, Codafen Continus*, Codant, Codis*, Diarrest*, Dimotane Co*, Feminax, Migraleve*, Nurofen Plus, Panadeine, Panadol Ultra*, Paracodal, Solpadeine*, Solpadol*, Syndol*, Terpoin*, Tylex*, Veganin*	Pain: 120–240 mg daily Cough: 45–120 mg daily Diarrhoea: 30–180 mg daily
co-dydramol* (mixture of dihydro-codeine and paracetamol)	Remedeine*	1–2 tablets 4–6 times daily (maximum 8 daily)
co-proxamol* (mixture of dextro-propoxyphene and paracetamol)	Cosalgesic*, Fortagesic*, Distalgesic*	2 tablets per dose (maximum 8 tablets daily)
dextromoramide	Palfium	5–20 mg daily
dextropropoxyphene	–	65 mg 3–4 times daily
diamorphine (heroin)	–	Given by injection in acute situations Orally for chronic pain: 5–10 mg 6 times daily
dihydrocodeine	DF118, DHC Continus, Drocode, Paracodin, Rikodeine	30 mg 4–6 times daily

dipipanone	Diconal	1–3 tablets 4 times daily
fentanyl	Duragesic ('25', '50', '75', '100'), Fentanyl, Sublimaze	1 patch applied (dose depends upon pain and previous use of opiates)
hydromorphone	Dilaudid, Palladone	1.3 mg 6 times daily, to increase as necessary
	Palladone SR	4 mg twice daily, to increase as necessary
levorphanol	Dromoran, Levo-Dromoran	2–3 mg 3 or 4 times daily
meptazinol	Meptid	200 mg 4–8 times daily
methadone	Dolophine, Methadose, Physeptone	5–10 mg 3–4 times daily
morphine	Anamorph, Kapanol, Morcap SR, Morphitec, M.O.S, MSIR, MS Contin, MST Continus, MXL, Oramorph, Oramorph SR, Ordine*, Roxanol, Roxanol SR, Sevredol, Statex, Zomorph	5–20 mg 6 times daily
pentazocine	Fortral, Sosenol, Talwin	50 mg 6–8 times daily
pethidine	–	50–150 mg 6 times daily
phenazocine	Narphen	5 mg 4–6 times daily
tramadol	Dromadol SR, Tramake Insts, Tramal, Ultram, Zamadol, Zamadol SR, Zydol, Zydol SR, Zydol XL	50–100 mg 6 times daily (maximum 400 mg daily)

Table 16.2: Morphine and its relatives

Uses: moderate to severe pain, cough in terminal illness

When not to be used: difficult breathing, asthma or chronic bronchitis, chronic lung disease, low blood pressure, liver disease, head injury, together with use of monoamine oxidase inhibitor antidepressants or within two weeks of stopping them

Cautions: elderly, hypothyroidism, kidney or liver impairment

Effects

General: sedation, weakness
Gastrointestinal: nausea, vomiting, constipation, abdominal pain, raised liver enzymes, jaundice
Musculoskeletal: muscle weakness
Central nervous system: dizziness, light-headedness, headache, convulsions
Psychological: euphoria, altered mood, hallucinations, psychosis
Skin: rash
Special senses: minor visual disturbances

Strength level: 2 (1 if taken symptomatically)

NEFOPAM

Generic name	Brand name	Dosage
nefopam	Acupan	90–270 mg daily

Table 16.3: Nefopam

Uses: pain reliever

When not to be used: epilepsy

Cautions: liver or kidney impairment, elderly, urinary retention

Effects

General: drowsiness
Cardiovascular: palpitations, rapid heart rate
Gastrointestinal: nausea, dry mouth, vomiting
Urogenital: urinary retention, colours the urine pink
Central nervous system: light-headedness, headache
Psychological: insomnia, hallucinations, nervousness, confusion
Skin: sweating
Special senses: blurred vision

Strength level: 2 (1 if taken symptomatically)

PARACETAMOL (ACETAMINOPHEN)

Generic name	Brand name	Dosage
co-methiamol* (mixture of paracetamol and methionine)	Paradote*	2 tablets 6 times daily (maximum 8 daily)
paracetamol (acetaminophen)	Anadin Extra*, Cosalgesic*, Distalgesic*, Fortagesic*, Kapake*, Paradote*, Remedeine*, Solpadol*, Tylex*	0.5–1 g 4–6 times daily (maximum 4 g daily)

Table 16.4: Paracetamol (acetaminophen)

Uses: mild to moderate pain, fever

When not to be used: for more than 10 days for pain relief (five days for children), for more than three days for fever

Cautions: high blood pressure, oedema, severe kidney or liver impairment (because of sodium content of tablets).

Some people are more sensitive to paracetamol's toxic effects on the liver. These include alcoholics, those receiving barbiturates, those who are chronically malnourished.

Effects
General: allergic reactions, swelling, weakness, fatigue
Respiratory: difficulty breathing
Gastrointestinal: jaundice, bleeding from the bowel, pancreatitis, liver damage, low blood sugar
Urogenital: blood in the urine, cloudy urine, sudden decrease in amount of urine, kidney damage
Musculoskeletal: flank or lower back pain
Central nervous system: light-headedness, tremor
Blood: changes in the blood
Skin: rash, bleeding into the skin

Strength level: 2 (1 if taken symptomatically)

HOLISTIC MANAGEMENT

Any pain reliever used regularly can damage the kidneys. This is particularly true in the elderly and in conditions where chronic pain is a feature. In addition, it is common that the kidneys may already be involved in the disease process (e.g. autoimmune disease such as rheumatoid arthritis).

Non-steroidal anti-inflammatory drugs (see page 44) can be considered to be similar in their actions to aspirin.

Morphine and its relatives have mental effects as well as relieving pain and these can lead to sedation, drowsiness, confusion in the elderly and withdrawal symptoms of anxiety, restlessness and insomnia.

The following opiates are listed in order of increasing strength:
- codeine phosphate
- dextropropoxyphene
- dihydrocodeine
- methadone
- phenazocine
- dextromoramide, dipipanone, levorphanol, morphine
- diamorphine

The other pain relievers, aspirin and paracetamol being the main examples, affect other areas. Aspirin has a predilection for the gastrointestinal tract, so indigestion, peptic ulceration and upper gastrointestinal haemorrhage can occur. Paracetamol damages the liver and overdosage can be fatal, due to liver cell death. Both drugs, used regularly, cause kidney damage and my opinion is that analgesics are a major cause of debility, ill health and kidney-related disease in the elderly. Low backache, frequent urination and nocturnal urination are common symptoms.

Holistic treatment needs to be directed at the painful condition whilst reducing the pain relievers, perhaps with the prescription of less powerful agents.

Although these drugs relieve pain, they do so to a variable degree. Musculoskeletal problems are particularly resistant. In the long term, of course, they lead to more pain, because of their depleting effect. This was the situation with the case history on page 167. Regular use of pain relievers had caused more frequent and more severe migraines.

17 PARKINSON'S DISEASE

Parkinson's disease is characterised by tremor, rigidity and slowness of movement. Conventional medicine sees the cause as being a chemical imbalance in the brain. Therefore, conventional drug-based treatment prescribes chemicals to try to restore the 'normal' state of affairs.

BENZHEXOL (TRIHEXYPHENIDYL) AND RELATIVES

Generic name	Brand name	Dosage
benzhexol (trihexyphenidyl)	Aparkane, Apo-Trihex, Artane, Broflex, Novohexidyl, Trihexane, Trihexy	5–15 mg daily
benztropine (benzatropine)	Apo-Cogentin, Bensylate, Cogentin	1–4 mg daily. (maximum 6 mg daily)
biperiden	Akineton	5–12 mg daily
orphenadrine	Biorphen, Disipal, Norflex, Phenrine	150–400 mg daily
procyclidine	Arpicolin, Kemadrin	2.5 mg 3 times daily to maximum of 30 mg daily

Table 17.1: Benzhexol (trihexyphenidyl) and relatives

Uses: Parkinson's disease, drug-induced Parkinson-like symptoms (not tardive dyskinesia)

When not to be used: enlarged prostate, pyloric stenosis, paralytic ileus, narrow-angle glaucoma

Cautions: hyperthyroidism, high blood pressure, heart, liver or kidney disorders, elderly, obstruction of the digestive or urinary systems. People on long-term treatment should be closely monitored.

Effects

General: nausea or nervousness is experienced by up to 50% of patients

Cardiovascular: flushing

Gastrointestinal: dry mouth, constipation, nausea, vomiting

Urogenital: difficult urination

Central nervous system: dizziness, tardive dyskinesia

Psychological: euphoria, confusion, agitation, delusions, hallucinations

Skin: dryness of skin, blurred vision

Special senses: glaucoma

Strength level: 2

LEVODOPA AND ITS RELATIVES

Generic name	Brand name	Dosage
amantadine	Antadine, Symadine, Symmetrel	100–200 mg daily
co-beneldopa	Madopar*, Madopar CR*	400–800 mg daily
co-careldopa	Sinemet* (62.5, 110 and Plus), Half Sinemet CR*, Sinemet CR*	Depends upon exact formulation
entacapone	Comtan, Comtess	200 mg–2 g daily
levodopa	Carbilev*, Dopar, Larodopa, Kinson*, Madopar*, Sinacarb, Sinemet*	125–500 mg daily
lysuride (lisuride)	Revanil	Up to 5 mg daily
pergolide	Celance, Permax	3 mg daily
pramipexole	Mirapex, Mirapexin	Up to 3.3 mg daily
ropinirole	Requip	3–9 mg daily (maximum 24 mg daily)
selegiline	Centrapryl, Eldepryl, Selgene, Stilline, Vivapryl, Zelapar	10 mg daily

Table 17.2: Levodopa and its relatives

Uses: Parkinson's disease

When not to be used: with monoamine oxidase inhibitor antidepressants (except low doses of selective monoamine oxidase B inhibitors), narrow-angle glaucoma, drug-induced Parkinson's disease-like symptoms

Cautions: severe heart, circulatory or lung disease, asthma, kidney or liver impairment, endocrine disease, history of stomach or duodenal ulcer, psychosis.

All patients must be carefully monitored for psychological changes such as mental disturbances, depression, suicidal ideas, behavioural changes.

Regular monitoring of liver, kidney and heart function are recommended during long-term therapy.

Effects

General: sleepiness, weakness, faintness, fatigue, malaise, hot flushes

Cardiovascular: palpitations, high blood pressure, low blood pressure (particularly on standing), chest pain, phlebitis, oedema

Respiratory: abnormal breathing patterns, breathlessness, hoarseness

Gastrointestinal: nausea, poor appetite, vomiting, gastrointestinal bleeding, duodenal ulcer, dry mouth, bitter taste, sialorrhoea, difficulty swallowing, teeth grinding, hiccoughs, abdominal pain, constipation, diarrhoea, flatulence, burning tongue, weight gain, weight loss

Urogenital: urinary retention, urinary incontinence, dark urine, priapism

Musculoskeletal: muscle twitching, muscle cramp

Central nervous system: numbness, involuntary movements, trismus, loss of balance, dizziness, pins and needles, hand tremor, spasmodic fixed deviation of eyes, headache, neuroleptic malignant syndrome, falling, abnormalities of posture and walking

Psychological: mental changes, paranoid ideas, psychosis, depression, suicidal tendencies, insomnia, nightmares, hallucinations, delusions, euphoria, confusion, agitation, anxiety, behavioural changes

Blood: reduction in white blood cell count that may lead to increased infections, anaemia with or without destruction of red blood cells, *low platelet* count leading to bleeding into the skin, prolonged bleeding after injury and spontaneous bruising, *severe acute reduction in numbers of neutrophils* (type of white blood cell) leading to severe bacterial infections that are usually fatal

Skin: sweating, dark sweat, rash, hair loss, malignant melanoma

Special senses: double vision, blurred vision, dilated pupils, involuntary closing of eyelids, Horner's syndrome

Strength level: 2

BROMOCRIPTINE AND ITS RELATIVES

Generic name	Brand name	Dosage
bromocriptine	Kripton, Parlodel	5–7.5 mg daily (maximum of 30 mg daily)
cabergoline	Cabaser, Dostinex	2–6 mg daily
quinagolide	Norprolac	75–150 mcg daily

Table 17.3: Bromocriptine and its relatives

Uses: suppression of lactation (not quinagolide), Parkinson's disease, benign breast disease, suppression of prolactin (some cases of infertility, breast milk secretion)

When not to be used: toxaemia of pregnancy, high blood pressure after childbirth

Cautions: in people with heart disease, stomach or duodenal ulcers or symptoms and/or a history of serious mental disorders.

Blood pressure should be carefully monitored, especially during the first days of treatment. Extra care should be taken in those who are taking or who have recently taken drugs that can alter blood pressure.

Gynaecological assessment, preferably including cervical and endometrial cell examination (cervical or PAP smear and D & C), is recommended for women having prolonged treatment. Assessment twice yearly is suggested for post-menopausal women and once yearly for women with regular menstruation.

Effects
General: pallor of the fingers and toes induced by cold, drowsiness
Cardiovascular: low blood pressure (particularly on standing)
Gastrointestinal: nausea, vomiting, mild constipation, dry mouth
Musculoskeletal: leg cramps
Central nervous system: dizziness, headache, involuntary movements
Psychological: excitation, hallucinations, confusion

Strength level: 2

HOLISTIC MANAGEMENT OF PARKINSON'S DISEASE

Drug treatment only helps relieve symptoms in the short term – there is no claim to cure – and side-effects are common. Patients with a marked degree of rigidity tend to become more mobile but develop an increase in tremor, while those with a marked degree of tremor tend to shake less but develop an increase in rigidity.

With long-term treatment, there may come a point where the drugs seem to be ineffective and only produce adverse effects, with anxiety, severely restricted movement and unsteadiness. Here the drugs may be given intermittently to regain some effectiveness.

There is increasing evidence that drugs may lead to acceleration of the disease. Drug withdrawal tends to lead to exacerbation of the tremor, rigidity and slow movement, depending on the individual case. Reduction in drug dosage must therefore be slow and should be judged according to the patient's symptoms. Response can be very good if people receive holistic medical treatment early enough. It is more difficult in chronic cases with long-term drug use. However, it can be very rewarding to treat people with Parkinson's disease, as small increases in function can have dramatic effects on quality of life. Reduction of drug dosage removes many of the side-effects, especially those of anxiety and insomnia. At the same time, treatment definitely strengthens people, so their original symptoms improve.

18 PSYCHOACTIVE DRUGS

Psychoactive drugs are used in the treatment of psychological disease. In addition, they are increasingly being used to remove some of the normal reactions we all experience in life – sadness, irritability, anxiety and so forth. Prozac is well known as a drug that is used to produce 'happy, shiny' people, but other psychoactive drugs are used to modify mood in people who certainly do not have a classified psychiatric disorder.

Such manipulation of our psychological state creates many difficulties. It leads people to believe that they can be mentally and emotionally balanced through the use of prescribed chemicals. Consequently, people are not encouraged to use their own resources and are disempowered from finding their own sources of support. Medical professionals frequently underplay the seriousness and frequency of addiction and the withdrawal symptoms that can occur when such medication is reduced or stopped.

ANTIDEPRESSANTS

There are three groups of drugs used in the treatment of depression. They are tricyclic antidepressants, monoamine oxidase inhibitors and the newer, selective serotonin re-uptake inhibitors, of which Prozac is the best-known example. There is little to choose between them in terms of safety and side-effects. They all sedate to some degree, although some may be prescribed with tranquillisers if there is anxiety with the depression. They may be given at night, because of their sedative actions.

Depression, in common with many psychological disorders, is conventionally thought to be due to a chemical imbalance within the brain. Antidepressants are often given in the hope that they will change the levels of these chemicals. In reality, there is no evidence that depression is caused by such a chemical balance or that antidepressants result in a 'balancing' of these chemicals. Such arguments are, however, frequently quoted as a justification for giving this medication.[1]

Depression is frequently merely a superficial emotion that is masking something deeper. The drugs only serve to give an improvement on a superficial level. They make no attempt at resolving or treating the underlying process; indeed this is now more likely to be ignored, because the person feels subjectively improved. In addition, the use of such medication reinforces the idea that there is little such patients can do themselves to change their situation or their emotional state.

In fact, depression is a loosely used term that can include many different emotions and it is essential to individualise the case. Some people are weepy, others have low mood with feelings of apathy, whilst others have feelings of sadness and grief. In conventional medicine, all people are given the same types of drug.

Monoamine oxidase inhibitors

Monoamine oxidase inhibitors are an older type of antidepressant and are used less frequently nowadays. Tricyclic antidepressants or Prozac and its clones have largely replaced them. They may be given for depression that does not respond to these other antidepressants or in cases of depression with physical manifestations such as paralysis or numbness (so-called 'hysteria').

Generic name	Brand name	Dosage
isocarbazid	–	30–60 mg daily
moclobemide	Arima, Aurorix, Manerix, Mohexal	150–600 mg daily
phenelzine	Nardil	15–30 mg 3 times daily
tranylcypromine	Parnate	10–30 mg daily

Table 18.1: Monoamine oxidase inhibitors

Uses: depression

When not to be used: liver damage or impairment, cerebrovascular disease.

These drugs should not be given within 14 days of taking tricyclic antidepressants.

Cautions: monoamine oxidase inhibitors interact with a wide range of medications, including opiate painkillers, adrenaline (epinephrine) and related drugs, amphetamines, dopamine, levodopa, blood pressure-lowering drugs, hypoglycaemic agents, anti-Parkinson drugs, local anaesthetics and central nervous system depressants (e.g. alcohol). They should be withdrawn two weeks before surgery or dentistry.

People taking these drugs should avoid cheese and foods containing tyramine, such as Oxo, Bovril, Marmite, during treatment and up to 14 days after ending treatment.

Patients should be told to restrict alcohol intake, to avoid heavy red wines and they should be warned about self-medication, especially with cold cures.

Great care must be taken in the elderly, those with agitation, evidence of cardiovascular disease, epilepsy, blood disorders, phaeochromocytoma, liver toxicity or diabetes mellitus.

Effects

General: severe hypertensive reactions (notably in association with foods containing tyramine), pain, substernal pain, pallor, flushing, weakness

Cardiovascular: palpitations, headache, rise in blood pressure, severe occipital headache, slow heart rate, rapid heart rate, abnormal heart rhythms, oedema, low blood pressure (especially when standing)

Gastrointestinal: nausea, vomiting, dry mouth, weight gain, increased appetite, raised liver enzymes

Urogenital: difficult urination

Musculoskeletal: stiff muscles

Central nervous system: headache, drowsiness, dizziness, peripheral neuropathy

Psychological: insomnia, restlessness, agitation, hypomania, hallucinations, anxiety

Blood: blood disorders

Skin: sweating, bleeding into the skin, rash

Special senses: dilated pupils, sensitivity of eyes to light, blurred vision

Strength level: 2

Tricyclic antidepressants

These are the most commonly used antidepressants, together with Prozac and its relatives.

Generic name	Brand name	Dosage
amitriptyline	Adepril, Amitrol, Domical, Elavil, Emitrip, Endep, Etrafon*, Lentizol, Levate, Limbitrol*, Novotriptyn, Saroten, Trepiline, Triavil*, Triptafen*, Tryptizol, Tryptanol	50–150 mg daily
amoxapine	Asendin, Asendis	100–300 mg daily
clomipramine	Anafranil, Anafranil SR, Placil	10–250 mg daily

desipramine	Norpramin, Pertofan, Pertofrane	100–150 mg daily (maximum dose 300 mg daily
dothiepin (dosulepin)	Dothapax, Dothep, Jardin, Prepadine, Prothiaden, Thaden	75–150 mg daily
doxepin	Adapin, Deptran, Sinequan, Triadaprin, Zonalon	75–300 mg daily
imipramine	Ethipramine, Impril, Janimine, Miprilin, Norfranil, Novapramine, Panpramine, Tipramine, Tofranil	75–200 mg daily Children: not recommended for depression but used for bedwetting; 7-year-olds: 25 mg daily; 8–11-year-olds: 25–50 mg daily; over 11: 50–75 mg daily (not to be used for longer than 3 months)
lofepramine	Emdalen, Gamanil	140–210 mg daily
maprotiline[2]	Ludiomil	25–150 mg daily
mianserin	Bolvidon, Lantanon, Lerivon, Lumin, Tolvon	30–90 mg daily
nortriptyline	Allegron, Aventyl, Motipress*, Motival*, Nortrilen, Pamelor	75–150 mg daily
protryptiline	Concordin, Vivactil	15–60 mg daily
trazodone	Desyrel, Molipaxin	150–300 mg daily
trimipramine	Apo-Trimip, Rhotrimine, Surmontil, Tydamine	50–300 mg daily

Table 18.2: Tricyclic antidepressants

Uses: depression, panic disorders, nerve pain, enuresis in children

When not to be used: together with the monoamine oxidase inhibitor antidepressants or within three weeks of stopping them, after a heart attack, irregular heart rhythms, mania, severe liver disease, children under the age of six, narrow angle glaucoma, retention of urine

Cautions: history of epilepsy, liver impairment, history of retention of urine, enlarged prostate, increased intra-ocular pressure, heart and circulatory disorders, hyperthyroidism, those taking thyroid medication or anticholinergic drugs.

The elderly are particularly susceptible to developing psychological effects.

Effects

General: hot flushes, fatigue, feelings of unrest, yawning, extremely high fever.
Withdrawal symptoms have been reported in up to 10% of patients following sudden withdrawal. These include nausea, vomiting, abdominal pain, diarrhoea, insomnia, headache, nervousness and anxiety.

Cardiovascular: low blood pressure (when standing), palpitations, rapid heart rate, increased blood pressure

Gastrointestinal: dry mouth, constipation, poor appetite, increased appetite, nausea, vomiting, abdominal disorders, diarrhoea, taste disturbance, raised liver enzymes, hepatitis, jaundice, weight gain

Urogenital: urinary disturbances, disturbances of libido and sexual potency

Musculoskeletal: muscle weakness, increased muscle tone

Central nervous system: dizziness, tremor, headache, muscle spasms, speech disorders, pins and needles, convulsions, EEG changes, loss of balance

Endocrine: antidiuretic hormone secretion syndrome

Women's health: secretion of milk from breasts, breast enlargement

Psychological: drowsiness, confusion, disorientation, anxiety, impaired memory, behavioural difficulties in children, hallucinations, agitation, sleep disturbances, mania, hypomania, aggressiveness, insomnia, nightmares, depression, poor concentration, depersonalisation, psychosis, worsening of psychosis

Blood: reduction in white blood cell count that may lead to increased infections, *severe acute reduction in numbers of neutrophils* (type of white blood cell) leading to severe bacterial infections that are usually fatal, *low platelet count* leading to bleeding into the skin, prolonged bleeding after injury and spontaneous bruising, *increase in numbers of eosinophils* (type of white blood cell) usually denoting allergic reaction, *reduction in numbers of red and white blood cells and platelets* leading to anaemia, increased risk of infection and spontaneous bruising/bleeding

Skin: sweating, allergic skin reactions, sensitivity to light, itching, bleeding into the skin

Special senses: difficulty focusing, blurred vision, glaucoma, tinnitus

Strength level: 2

Selective serotonin re-uptake inhibitors (SSRIs)

Selective serotonin re-uptake inhibitors are the flavour of the month amongst medical practitioners. They have powerful effects and, despite all protestations to the contrary, are clearly addictive and produce withdrawal symptoms when they are stopped.

Generic name	Brand name	Dosage
citalopram	Celexa, Cipramil, Prisdal, Seropram	20–80 mg daily
fluoxetine	Deprax, Erocap, Eufor, Lorien, Lovan, Prozac, Psiquial, Veritina, Zactin	20–60 mg daily
fluvoxamine	Faverin, Luvox, Maveral	100–300 mg daily
paroxetine	Aropax, Lumin, Paxil, Seroxat	20–50 mg daily
sertraline	Lustral, Sercerin, Tolrest, Zoloft	50–200 mg daily (more than 150 mg daily should not be taken for more than 8 weeks)

Table 18.3: Selective serotonin re-uptake inhibitors (SSRIs)

Uses: depression, obsessive-compulsive disorder, bulimia nervosa, psychological symptoms in the pre-menstrual phase

When not to be used: unstable epilepsy, severe kidney failure. Not to be taken within 2 weeks of stopping treatment with monoamine oxidase inhibitor antidepressants.

Cautions: convulsions occur in approximately 0.2%, therefore patients with epilepsy should be carefully monitored. Patients who are given electroconvulsive treatment at the same time as these drugs are at risk of developing prolonged convulsions.

A lower dose is necessary in those with liver disease or mild/moderate kidney failure.

Patients with diabetes mellitus taking hypoglycaemic drugs such as insulin may need to reduce their dosage.

Effects
General: weakness, fever, fatigue
Cardiovascular: low blood pressure (particularly on standing), high blood pressure,

palpitations, rapid heart rate, irregular heart rates which can be life-threatening
Respiratory: sore throat, breathlessness, pneumonia
Gastrointestinal: nausea, diarrhoea, dry mouth, appetite loss, indigestion, raised
liver enzymes, vomiting, bleeding from the bowel and stomach, pancreatitis
Urogenital: decreased libido, sexual dysfunction, raised serum urea, vaginal
bleeding after drug withdrawal
Musculoskeletal: joint pain, muscle pain
Central nervous system: headache, tremor, dizziness, convulsions, confusion,
involuntary movements, buccal-lingual-masticatory syndrome, neuroleptic
malignant syndrome-like symptoms, stroke, movement disorders, worsening of
pre-existing movement disorders
Endocrine: raised serum prolactin levels, low blood sugar
Psychological: insomnia, hallucinations, psychosis, hypomania, mania, suicidal
ideas, violent behaviour, mood changes, nervousness, drowsiness, anxiety
Blood: reduction in numbers of red and white blood cells and platelets leading to
anaemia, increased risk of infection and spontaneous bruising/bleeding, *low
platelet count* leading to bleeding into the skin, prolonged bleeding after injury and
spontaneous bruising, *reduced white cell counts, anaemia* due to destruction of red
blood cells
Skin: sweating, rash, acne, bleeding into the skin
Special senses: visual disturbances, photophobia

Strength level: 2

Mirtazepine

Generic name	Brand name	Dosage
mirtazepine	Remeron, Zispin	20–80 mg daily

Table 18.4: Mirtazepine

Uses: depression

Cautions: bone marrow depression, due to its ability to damage blood-forming cells.
Any symptoms such as fever, sore throat, sore mouth or other signs of infection
require stopping treatment and taking a blood count.

Regular and close monitoring should be performed in people with epilepsy, liver and
kidney impairment, heart diseases such as recent heart attack, angina pectoris, low
blood pressure and abnormal heart rhythms, urinary disturbances such as enlarged
prostate, narrow-angle glaucoma and diabetes mellitus.

Effects

Cardiovascular: low blood pressure, oedema
Gastrointestinal: weight gain, raised liver enzymes
Central nervous system: convulsions, tremor, muscle spasms
Psychological: mania
Blood: bone marrow depression, increase in numbers of eosinophils (type of white blood cell) usually denoting allergic reaction, *reduction in numbers of granulocytes* (type of white blood cell), *severe acute reduction in numbers of neutrophils* (type of white blood cell) leading to severe bacterial infections that are usually fatal, *reduction in numbers of red and white blood cells and platelets* leading to anaemia, increased risk of infection and bleeding into the skin, prolonged bleeding after injury and spontaneous bruising, *low platelet count* leading to bleeding into the skin, prolonged bleeding after injury and spontaneous bruising
Skin: rash

Strength level: 2

Nefazodone

Generic name	Brand name	Dosage
nefazodone	Dutonin, Nefadar, Serzone	50–300 mg twice daily

Table 18.5: Nefazodone

Uses: depression

Cautions: liver or kidney impairment, epilepsy, recent heart attack, unstable heart disease, history of mania or hypomania

Effects

General: weakness, somnolence, chills, fever
Cardiovascular: low blood pressure (particularly on standing), vasodilatation, fainting
Gastrointestinal: dry mouth, nausea, constipation, diarrhoea, vomiting, raised liver enzymes, hepatitis, liver failure, liver damage
Urogenital: priapism
Musculoskeletal: joint pains
Central nervous system: dizziness, poor co-ordination, light-headedness, pins and needles, headache, loss of balance
Psychological: abnormal dreams, hallucinations, mania, hypomania, anxiety, poor memory, confusion

Skin: rash, sweating
Special senses: blurred vision, other visual disturbances

Strength level: 2

Reboxetine

Generic name	Brand name	Dosage
reboxetine	Edronax, Norebox, Vestra	4–6 mg twice daily

Table 18.6: Reboxetine

Uses: depression

Cautions: history of convulsions, retention of urine, enlarged prostate, glaucoma, history of heart disease when used with drugs that lower blood pressure

Effects
Cardiovascular: palpitations, rapid heart rate, low blood pressure
Gastrointestinal: dry mouth, constipation
Urogenital: impotence, urinary tract infection, painful urination, urinary hesitancy or retention
Central nervous system: dizziness, pins and needles, vertigo, convulsions (requires stopping treatment)
Psychological: insomnia, mania, hypomania
Skin: sweating

Strength level: 2

Tryptophan

Generic name	Brand name	Dosage
tryptophan	Optimax	2 tablets 3 times daily

Table 18.7: Tryptophan

Uses: depression

Cautions: when used with monoamine oxidase inhibitor antidepressants, as their side-effects may be increased. When taken together with chlorpromazine or its relatives (see page 202) or benzodiazepines (see page 195), there may be sexual disinhibition.

Effects

>*General:* drowsiness
>*Gastrointestinal:* nausea
>*Central nervous system:* headache, light-headedness

Strength level: 2

Venlafaxine

Generic name	Brand name	Dosage
venlafaxine	Dobupal, Efexor	75–150 mg daily

Table 18.8: Venlafaxine

Uses: depression

Cautions: risk of suicide, convulsions (or a history of convulsions), heart attack, unstable heart disease, kidney impairment, liver cirrhosis

Effects

>*General:* weakness, chills, fatigue, sleepiness
>*Cardiovascular:* flushing, high blood pressure, palpitations, low blood pressure (particularly on standing), raised serum cholesterol, low serum sodium
>*Gastrointestinal:* nausea, dry mouth, constipation, poor appetite, indigestion, abdominal pain, vomiting, weight gain, raised liver enzymes, diarrhoea
>*Urogenital:* impotence, abnormal ejaculatory orgasm, decreased libido
>*Central nervous system:* headache, dizziness, nervousness, anxiety, tremor, pins and needles, confusion, vertigo
>*Psychological:* insomnia, agitation
>*Skin:* sweating
>*Special senses:* blurred vision

Strength level: 2

Holistic management

These medications are all very powerful agents. It can be seen from the list of effects that antidepressants heat up the body and have similar effects to amphetamines ('speed'). They are 'uppers' or stimulants and may be effective in lifting the black mood of depression. They cause agitation, restlessness and, in severe cases, psychosis. They burn up the patient, leading to constipation, dryness of mouth, blurred vision and so on.

They are, conventionally, given for at least three weeks, because it is considered that it takes that long for an effect to begin. This is not always true, as, in some people, the mood changes after a few days. Withdrawal of these drugs leads to the appearance of depression, low mood, perhaps with weeping and sighing. Typical withdrawal symptoms include nausea, headache, malaise, irritability, restlessness, dreams and other sleep disturbances. Sudden cessation of these drugs can lead to severe difficulties and must be avoided if at all possible.

Any drug reduction must be slow to enable time to be taken dealing with the released symptoms. Appropriate help such as psychological support, counselling, or psychotherapy may be required to help with the deeper emotional states.

Case history

A woman aged 40 presented for treatment with depression and anxiety, which she had experienced for the previous 15 years. The symptoms would come and go. There was also tiredness, frequent sweating (particularly at night), feelings of tension in the stomach. She described herself as a tense kind of person and lacking in confidence. Her sleep was good, but she sometimes woke in the night at 2 a.m. She experienced occasional palpitations.

Medication
Prothiaden: 75 mg, 3 tablets at night
Pulse: thin and floating on left
Tongue: red, dry, paler edges

Diagnosis: Kidney and Heart Yin Deficiency, Liver Yin and Blood Deficiency
Treatment principles: nourish Kidney and Heart Yin, nourish Liver Yin and Blood
Acupuncture treatment: **H-6** Tongli, **K-6** Zhaohai, **P-6** Neiguan, **K-3** Taixi

Chinese herbal formula
Dang Shen *Radix Codonopsis Pilosulae* 9 g
Huang Qi *Radix Astragali* 6 g
Dang Gui *Radix Angelicae Sinensis* 6 g
Zhi Gan Cao *Radix Glycyrrhizae Uralensis* (Honey fried) 3 g
Suan Zao Ren *Semen Ziziphi Spinosae* 9 g
Yuan Zhi *Radix Polygalae Tenuifoliae* 5 g
Sheng Jiang *Cortex Zingiberis Officinalis Recens* 5 g
Da Zao *Fructus Zizyphi Jujubae* 5 g
Chen Pi *Pericarpium Citri Reticulatae* 5 g
Lian Zi *Semen Nelumbinis Nuciferae* 8 g
Fu Shen *Sclerotium Poriae Cocos Pararadicis* 6 g

Outcome

At her second visit, one month later, she had had some relief, with no anxiety, for the previous two weeks. She found that practising breathing relaxation helped her. At visit three, six weeks later, she had experienced one mild episode of depression with anxiety but this had passed off easily. At her fourth visit, three weeks later, she had continued to improve and had more energy. She reduced the Prothiaden to two at night.

At visit five, four weeks later, she was good and felt well. She reduced the Prothiaden further to one at night. At the sixth visit, four weeks later, she again felt well and decided to stop the Prothiaden. She experienced some irritability and frustration in the following four weeks, but this settled well and she remains drug free five years later.

This is a situation where the diagnosis is clear and treatment can begin. It is important not to interfere with the medication until an improvement is seen. We only discussed reducing the medication at the fourth visit. The next visit will give useful information about how quickly or slowly reduction can proceed. She was well, with no significant flare-ups, so her dosage was reduced again. She was able to reduce her dosage monthly until she was drug free some 21 weeks after beginning treatment. It is significant that she developed some irritability and frustration after this last drug dosage was stopped. Such releases of suppressions are common. Too rapid a drug withdrawal may lead to the strong release of suppressed feelings. It is better to deal with these before further drug reduction takes place.

'MINOR' TRANQUILLISERS (ANXIOLYTICS)

Tranquillisers are divided into two groups, according to the severity of action and their indications. The 'major' tranquillisers are used for the treatment of psychotic disorders such as schizophrenia (see page 200).

The 'minor' tranquillisers are commonly used to treat insomnia and anxiety. They relieve the subjective feelings of anxiety, restlessness and insomnia. There is no essential difference between those given for anxiety and those given for insomnia (hypnotics). Women are prescribed them much more commonly than men, as one would expect in view of the more frequent (mis)diagnosis of neurosis and hysteria in females. They rapidly cause dependence and addiction. They can be difficult to stop, even after a short period of use. Withdrawal symptoms such as anxiety, difficulty sleeping and restlessness are common and may be experienced after two weeks. Increased sensitivity to external stimuli, particularly sound, is a common withdrawal symptom also. Such withdrawal symptoms can become so severe that psychotic features appear, with behavioural disturbances and delusional symptoms.

The most frequently used drugs are benzodiazepines, a common example of which is Valium. There is a move in some quarters to use antidepressants, betablockers or 'major' tranquillisers for anxiety, because of the increasingly recognised danger of dependence with benzodiazepines. This is a recipe for disaster. These drugs are also addictive and more powerful, and therefore more hazardous.

It is important that any dosage reduction is slow. This may mean reducing the amount of drug by a tiny fraction each time. The support of family, friends and self-help programmes is invaluable, but the major source of help for the symptoms is from effective treatment by holistic medicine. Acupuncture and homoeopathy have proven track records in helping such patients. As the patient becomes stronger, the process becomes easier.

Benzodiazepines

Generic name	Brand name	Dosage
alprazolam	Alprox Tablets, Alzam, Apo-Alpraz, Kalma, Novo Alprazol, Ralozam, Xanax	0.5–4 mg daily
bromazepam	Brazepam, Lectopam, Lexomyl, Lexotan, Lexotanil	3–18 mg daily
chlordiazepoxide	Libritabs, Librium, Lipoxide, Novopoxide, Solium, Tropium	10–100 mg daily
clonazepam	Klonopin, Paxam, Rivotril	4–8 mg daily
clorazepate	Gen-XENE, Novoclopate, Tranxene	7.5–22.5 mg daily
diazepam	Antenex, Anxicalm, Atensine, Benzopin, Dialar, Diazemuls, Ducene, Novodipam, Pax, Propam, Rimapam, Stesolid, Tensium, Valclair, Valium, Vazepam, Vivol	Anxiety: 6–30 mg daily Muscle spasm: 2–60 mg daily
estazolam	ProSom	1–2 mg at bedtime
flunitrazepam	Hypnodorm, Hypnor, Insom, Novolorazem, Nu-Loraz, Rohypnol	0.5–1 mg

flurazepam	Dalmane, Durapam, Novoflupam, Somno	15–30 mg at bedtime
halazepam	Paxipam	20–40 mg 3 or 4 times daily
loprazolam	Dormonoct	1–2 mg at bedtime
lorazepam	Alzapam, Ativan, Temesta, Tranqipam	1–4 mg daily
lormetazepam	Loramet	0.5–1.5 mg at bedtime
nitrazepam	Alodorm, Arem, Mogadon, Ormodon, Remnos, Somnipar, Somnite, Unisomnia	2.5–10 mg at bedtime
oxazepam	Alepam, Medopam, Murelax, Purata, Serax, Serenid, Serepax, Seresta, Zapex	Anxiety: 10–30 mg 3–4 times daily. Insomnia: 15–25 mg (maximum 50 mg) at bedtime
prazepam	Centrax, Demetrin, Verstran	10–60 mg daily
quazepam	Doral, Dormé	7.5–15 mg at bedtime
temazepam	Euhypnos Elixir, Nocturne, Nomapam, Normison, Restoril, Razepam, Temaze, Temtabs, Tenox, Z-Pam	10–60 mg daily
triazolam	Halcion	0.125–0.25 mg at night

Table 18.9: Benzodiazepines

Uses: insomnia, anxiety

When not to be used: breathing difficulties, sleep apnoea syndrome, obsessional states, psychosis and myasthenia gravis. They should not be used on their own in depression or in anxiety with depression.

Cautions: lung disease, muscle weakness, history of drug or alcohol abuse, marked personality disorder, porphyria.

The dose should be reduced in the elderly, in patients who are weak and in liver or kidney impairment.

They should not be used for a long time (more than three weeks) and withdrawal must always be slow.

Effects

General: drowsiness, dependence, pain, tiredness, lethargy, increased risk of accidents, increased risk of falling

Cardiovascular: low blood pressure, thrombophlebitis

Respiratory: breathing difficulties

Gastrointestinal: nausea, salivation changes, increased appetite, weight gain, gastrointestinal disturbances, jaundice, raised liver enzymes

Urogenital: changes in libido, incontinence, urinary retention

Musculoskeletal: muscle weakness, joint pain

Central nervous system: headache, vertigo, tremor, loss of balance, light-headedness, dizziness, slurred speech, stammering, poor co-ordination

Women's health: menstrual symptoms, sexual problems

Psychological: aggression, mood swings, lack of motivation, personality change, anxiety, irritability, difficulty sleeping, dream-disturbed sleep, confusion, poor memory, poor concentration, relaxation, feelings of isolation, depression, over-sedation, impaired judgement, difficulty thinking clearly

Blood: blood disorders

Skin: rash

Special senses: blurred vision, double vision

Strength level: 2

Buspirone

Generic name	Brand name	Dosage
buspirone	Buspar	15–30 mg daily (maximum 45 mg daily)

Table 18.10: Buspirone

Uses: anxiety

When not to be used: epilepsy, severe kidney or liver impairment

Cautions: Parkinson's disease or possibility of developing it, history of liver or kidney impairment. People with kidney or liver impairment should be closely monitored with regular kidney and liver function tests.

Effects

General: drowsiness, fatigue

Cardiovascular: rapid heart rate, palpitations, chest pain
Gastrointestinal: nausea, diarrhoea, dry mouth
Central nervous system: dizziness, headache, light-headedness
Psychological: excitement, confusion, nervousness
Skin: sweating, clamminess

Strength level: 2

Zolpidem

Generic name	Brand name	Dosage
zolpidem	Ambien, Stilnoct, Stilnox	10 mg at bedtime

Table 18.11: Zolpidem

Uses: insomnia

When not to be used: sleep apnoea, myasthenia gravis, severe liver impairment, acute breathlessness, lung disease, psychotic illness

Cautions: depression

Effects
General: drowsiness, fatigue
Gastrointestinal: gastrointestinal disturbances
Urogenital: changes in libido
Musculoskeletal: muscle weakness, loss of balance
Central nervous system: headache, dizziness
Psychological: inappropriate behaviour, depression, restlessness, agitation, irritability, aggression, rages, delusions, nightmares, hallucinations, psychoses, numbed emotions, poor concentration, confusion, loss of memory, suicidal tendencies
Skin: skin reactions
Special senses: double vision

Strength level: 2

Zopiclone

Generic name	Brand name	Dosage
zopiclone	Imovane, Zimovane	3.75–7.5 mg

Table 18.12: Zopiclone

Uses: insomnia

When not to be used: myasthenia gravis, respiratory failure, sleep apnoea syndrome, severe liver impairment

Cautions: liver and kidney impairment, the elderly, history of drug abuse, psychiatric illness. Not to be used for a long period of time (longer than three weeks) and withdrawal must be slow.

Effects

General: drowsiness, allergic reactions

Gastrointestinal: metallic or bitter taste, gastrointestinal disturbances, nausea, vomiting, dry mouth

Central nervous system: dizziness, light-headedness, lack of co-ordination, headache

Psychological: confusion, irritability, depression, hallucinations, nightmares, behavioural disturbances, aggression, loss of memory

Skin: nettle rash, rashes

Strength level: 2

Zaleplon

Generic name	Brand name	Dosage
zaleplon	Sonata	10 mg at bedtime

Table 18.13: Zaleplon

Uses: insomnia

When not to be used: sleep apnoea syndrome, myasthenia gravis, psychosis, severe lung or liver disease

Cautions: lung disease, breathing difficulties, liver impairment, history of drug or alcohol abuse. Not to be used for a long period of time (longer than three weeks) and withdrawal must be slow.

Effects

General: weakness, drowsiness
Central nervous system: headache, dizziness
Psychological: aggression, excitement, amnesia

Strength level: 2

'MAJOR' TRANQUILLISERS [3]

These tranquillisers are used to treat mental disturbances that are characterised by thought disorders, hallucinations and delusions. They are frequently classified as antipsychotic drugs, which has been described as one of the greatest marketing successes for psychiatric medication. This name implies that they work to suppress psychotic symptoms, which of course they do, but they do so by suppressing all mental functions, leading to marked symptoms of sedation. Their long-term effect is of damage to the structure of the brain, as is also seen in electroconvulsive treatment (ECT), and, in the case of 'major' tranquillisers, this is responsible for the development of tardive dyskinesia in up to 70% of patients.

The 'major' tranquillisers include the phenothiazines, of which the best-known example is Largactil. Newer varieties have come onto the market in the last few years that are reputed to have fewer side-effects. It is too early to tell if this is the case or not, but, historically, all drugs used for such conditions carry severe side-effects. These drugs lead to many problems because of their powerful action, and their use reflects the difficulties which current society has with such symptoms.

Tardive dyskinesia is a problem with this whole range of drugs. It is characterised by irregular repetitive involuntary movements, usually of the tongue and facial muscles. The trunk or limbs can also be affected. It is seen particularly in the elderly and in women. There are rhythmical involuntary movements of the tongue, face, mouth and jaw (e.g. protrusion of tongue, puffing of cheeks, puckering of mouth, chewing movements). There is no known effective treatment. It is generally irreversible. It can be worsened or precipitated by giving anti-Parkinson's disease drugs. Short-term involuntary movements can be seen after abrupt withdrawal of the drugs. Treatment by holistic medicine is also difficult, because the syndrome is the result of structural damage to the central nervous system.

Increased prolactin levels are common with this group of drugs. About one-third of human breast cancers are prolactin-dependent, and this must be taken into account before these drugs are prescribed.

Neuroleptic malignant syndrome (NMS)[4] is a recognised effect of all drugs that are used to treat psychotic conditions such as schizophrenia. NMS was first described in the 1960s, although the older-style treatments for schizophrenia (such as 'insulin shock therapy') also caused severe and sometimes fatal reactions. Some 0.2% of patients receiving neuroleptics develop this syndrome. The appearance of symptoms requires immediate cessation of drug treatment and it must never be restarted. Symptoms include rapid heart rate, sweating, rigidity, tremors, fever and changes in the patient's mental state that can lead to coma or catatonic states.

Sudden unexplained death is, of course, the ultimate side-effect of this class of drugs. This is almost certainly due to its effects on the heart and circulation. These drugs have effects on the ECG (EKG) of prolonging the QT interval. Therefore, they should not be used in those with low potassium levels or at the same time as drugs that also have this effect. These include other 'major' tranquillisers, tricyclic antidepressants, some antimalarial drugs, drugs for abnormal heart rhythms and some antihistamines. They should also not be used in people with a history of abnormal heart rhythms. Although these ECG changes may be of uncertain significance in conventional medicine, they clearly show that these drugs do affect heart function and the recognised side-effects of palpitations and heart rhythm abnormalities are further confirmation of serious effects upon this essential organ.

The conventional medical aim of treatment with these drugs is to control the symptoms of the psychosis, so there are no hard and fast rules about the ideal dosage. My opinion is that in most cases it is preferable to use the lowest dose possible that controls the symptoms. There is clearly room here for practitioners of holistic medicine to offer help in an appropriate set-up, as it is preferable for the patient to be treated in an environment with emotional and psychological support and access to professional psychotherapy or counselling.[5] It is not advisable to reduce medication, unless the patient is well motivated and has received holistic treatment for some time.

In some cases, these drugs can be further reduced in dosage as improvement occurs, or withdrawn if appropriate in carefully selected cases. It is clearly preferable to prevent the reappearance of the symptoms of delusion, hallucination, thought disorders and the like that occur in some cases of schizophrenia and related disorders. Therefore, reduction must always be slow and after some period of holistic treatment and psychological support. I have treated and continue to treat people with schizophrenia and other psychoses. Treatment is definitely helpful in moderating side-effects.

Chlorpromazine and its relatives

Generic name	Brand name	Dosage
chlorpromazine	Chloractil, Largactil, Ormazine, Taractan, Tarasan, Thorazine	Psychoses: 75–300 mg daily (maximum 1 g daily) Nausea and vomiting: 40–150 mg daily
flupenthixol (flupentixol)	Depixol, Fluanxol, Fluanxol Depot*	Psychoses: 3–9 mg daily (maximum 18 mg daily) Depression: 1–3 mg daily (maximum 2 mg daily in elderly)
fluphenazine	Anatensol, Modecate, Moditen, Motipress*, Motival*, Permitil, Prolixin	2.5–20 mg daily
methotrimeprazine (levomepromazine)	Levoprome, Nozinan	25–50 mg daily (maximum 1 g daily)
loxapine	Doxalin, Loxitane, Lozapac	60–100 mg daily (maximum 250 mg daily)
mesoridazine	Serentil	100–400 mg daily
oxypertine	–	80–120 mg daily (maximum 300 mg daily)
pericyazine	Neulactil, Neuleptil	75 mg daily (maximum 300 mg daily)
perphenazine	Etrafon*, Fentazin, Mutabon D*, Triavil*, Trilafon*, Triptafen*	4 mg 3 times daily (maximum 24 mg daily)
prochlorperazine	Buccastem, Compazine, Cotranzine, Mitil, Prorazin, Stemetil, Ultrazine, Vertigon	Psychoses: 75–100 mg daily Nausea, vomiting: 10 mg 2–3 times daily

promazine	Primazine, Prozine-50, Sparine	100–200 mg 4 times daily
sulpiride	Dolmatil, Eglonyl, Espiride, Sulparex, Sulpitil, Synconorm	200–400 mg twice daily (maximum 2.4 g daily)
thioridazine	Aldazine, Melleril, Melzine, Novo-Ridazine, Rideril, Ridazine	30–800 mg daily
trifluoperazine	Buccastem, Parstelin*, Solazine, Stelazine, Suprazine, Terfluzine, Vesprin	5 mg twice daily
zuclopenthixol	Acuphase, Clopixol, Clopixol Depot*	20–30 mg daily (maximum 150 mg daily)

Table 18.14: Chlorpromazine and its relatives

Uses: schizophrenia and other psychoses, mania, severe anxiety

When not to be used: coma caused by drugs such as alcohol, barbiturates or opiate pain relievers. Not to be used when taking drugs that affect the blood.

Caution: history of jaundice, liver impairment, blood disorders, heart disease, the elderly, very cold or very hot weather.

In long-term treatment, there must be regular monitoring, particularly for eye changes, blood counts, liver function tests and abnormal heart rhythms.

Effects
   General: sedation, sudden unexpected death, fever
   Cardiovascular: low blood pressure (particularly on standing), palpitations, rapid heart rate, serious heart rhythm abnormalities that can be fatal
   Respiratory: hyperventilation
   Gastrointestinal: dry mouth, jaundice
   Urogenital: failure of ejaculation
   Central nervous system: worsening of the symptoms of Parkinson's disease, physical restlessness, muscle spasms of neck, shoulders and trunk leading to abnormal postures

Endocrine: breast enlargement in men
Women's health: secretion of milk from breasts, no periods
Psychological: insomnia, agitation
Blood: raised ESR, increase in number of white blood cells, reduction in white blood cell count that may lead to increased infections, *severe acute reduction in numbers of neutrophils* (type of white blood cell) leading to severe bacterial infections that are usually fatal
Skin: sensitivity to light, rash, metallic greyish-mauve discoloration of exposed skin
Special senses: visual disturbances, eye changes

Strength level: 4

Haloperidol and its relatives

Generic name	Brand name	Dosage
benperidol	Anquil	0.25–1.5 mg daily
droperidol	Droleptan, Inapsin	5–20 mg 3–6 times daily
haloperidol	Cereen, Dozic, Fortunan, Haldol, Serenace	Mental illness: 1.5–20 mg daily initially (maximum 200 mg daily) Severe anxiety: 1 mg daily

Table 18.15: Haloperidol and its relatives

Uses: schizophrenia and other psychoses, violent behaviour, mania, agitation and restlessness

When not to be used: coma, sedation, depression

Cautions: Parkinson's disease or similar symptoms, hyperthyroidism, kidney failure, disease of the heart or circulation, epilepsy or convulsions.

Withdrawal symptoms include nausea, vomiting and insomnia and tardive dyskinesia (after sudden withdrawal).

In long-term treatment, there must be regular blood counts and liver and kidney function tests.

Effects

General: fever, sudden unexplained death, allergic reactions

Cardiovascular: unstable blood pressure, low blood pressure, palpitations, rapid heart rate, oedema

Gastrointestinal: nausea, vomiting, loss of appetite, constipation, indigestion, jaundice, raised liver enzymes, weight changes, excessive salivation

Musculoskeletal: muscle rigidity, elevated creatine phosphokinase (CPK) levels

Central nervous system: Parkinson's disease-like symptoms, muscle spasms of neck, shoulders and trunk leading to abnormal postures, rigidity, tremor, physically restless, spasmodic fixed deviation of eyes, laryngeal spasm, tardive dyskinesia (may be brought on or worsened by the use of drugs for Parkinson's disease), neuroleptic malignant syndrome, dizziness, headache, convulsions

Endocrine: raised serum prolactin levels, breast enlargement in men

Women's health: scanty or no periods, secretion of milk from breasts

Psychological: mentally dulled or slowed down, excitement, agitation, depression, altered consciousness, coma, confusion, insomnia

Blood: reduction in numbers of granulocytes (type of white blood cell)

Skin: sweating, rash, itching

Strength level: 4

Clozapine and its relatives

Generic name	Brand name	Dosage
clozapine	Clopine, Clozaril	25–900 mg daily
loxapine	Loxapac, Loxitane	20–100 mg daily

Table 18.16: Clozapine and its relatives

Uses: schizophrenia in those not responding to other drugs

When not to be used: coma, depression, history of drug-induced reduction of neutrophils (type of white blood cell) or agranulocytosis (severe acute reduction in numbers of neutrophils), bone marrow disorders, uncontrolled epilepsy, psychoses due to alcohol or drugs, drug intoxication, heart failure, sedation, severe kidney failure, liver disease, liver failure

Cautions: epilepsy, disease of the heart or circulation, glaucoma, retention of urine, enlargement of the prostate, narrow-angle glaucoma, paralysis of the intestines.

Before treatment, a total and differential white blood cell count must be done. Only people with normal results should receive the drug. During treatment, the total and differential white blood cell count must be done weekly for the first 18 weeks and at least two-weekly for the first year of treatment. When the patient has had treatment for one year with stable neutrophil counts, then monitoring may be changed to four-weekly intervals. Monitoring must continue for the duration of the treatment and for four weeks after cessation. The count must be checked immediately if there is sore throat, fever, flu-like symptoms or other symptoms suggestive of infection.

Liver function tests should be performed regularly in those with liver impairment.

The temperature may temporarily rise above 38°C at the beginning of treatment, usually within the first three weeks of treatment.

Effects

General: fatigue, drowsiness, sedation, fevers, sudden unexplained death

Cardiovascular: palpitations, rapid heart rate, low blood pressure (particularly on standing), high blood pressure, severe circulatory collapse, pericarditis, inflammation of heart muscle, heart failure, symptoms suggestive of heart attack, pericarditis, thrombosis, embolism

Respiratory: respiratory depression or arrest

Gastrointestinal: dry mouth, increased salivation, nausea, vomiting, constipation (which can be severe and complete), paralytic ileus, raised liver enzymes, hepatitis, jaundice, severe liver damage, difficulty swallowing, pancreatitis, raised blood sugar levels, marked weight gain with long-term treatment

Urogenital: incontinence, retention of urine, priapism, nephritis

Central nervous system: dizziness, headache, muscle spasms, convulsions, tremor, physical restlessness, rigidity, tardive dyskinesia, neuroleptic malignant syndrome, disturbances in sweating and temperature regulation

Blood: reduction of neutrophils (type of white blood cell) leading to increased susceptibility to infection, *severe acute reduction in numbers of neutrophils* (type of white blood cell) leading to severe bacterial infections which can prove fatal, *increase in number of white blood cells, increase in numbers of eosinophils* (type of white blood cell) usually denoting allergic reaction

Special senses: blurred vision

Strength level: 4

Molindone

Generic name	Brand name	Dosage
molindone	Lidone, Moban	5–25 mg 3 or 4 times daily (maximum 225 mg daily)

Table 18.17: Molindone

Uses: schizophrenia

When not to be used: avoid very hot environments (e.g. saunas), as this drug reduces sweating and therefore the ability to keep cool

Cautions: heart or circulatory disease, history of liver, thyroid or kidney problems, brain tumour, intestinal blockage.

Difficult urination, enlarged prostate, glaucoma, liver disease, Parkinson's disease, epilepsy and asthma may all worsen when taking this medication.

Effects
General: lethargy, sleepiness, weakness, drowsiness, fever, pallor
Cardiovascular: low blood pressure, high blood pressure, rapid heart rate, irregular heart rate, palpitations
Respiratory: stuffy nose, difficulty breathing
Gastrointestinal: dry mouth, constipation, weight gain, nausea, excessive salivation, raised liver enzymes, jaundice
Urogenital: difficult urination, sexual problems, reduced urination, increased sexual desire
Musculoskeletal: severe muscle stiffness, rigidity, stooped posture, muscle spasms
Central nervous system: headache, dizziness, light-headedness, convulsions, tremors, tardive dyskinesia, involuntary facial/tongue movements, involuntary movements of the arms or legs, trembling of limbs, shaking of the hands
Endocrine: breast enlargement in men, decreased libido
Women's health: menstrual irregularities, discharge of milk from the breast, decreased libido, breast enlargement
Psychological: restlessness, mental depression, unusual feeling of wellbeing (euphoria), hyperactivity, confusion
Blood: reduction in white blood cell count that may lead to increased infections
Skin: decreased sweating, increased sweating, rash
Special senses: blurred vision

Strength level: 4

Pimozide

Generic name	Brand name	Dosage
pimozide	Orap	2–20 mg daily

Table 18.18: Pimozide

Uses: schizophrenia

When not to be used: history of abnormal heart rhythms, sedation, depression, Parkinson's disease, at the same time as drugs that cause fluid or salt disturbances (e.g. diuretics)

Cautions: hyperthyroidism, liver disease, kidney failure, phaeochromocytoma, epilepsy, conditions predisposing to epilepsy (e.g. alcohol withdrawal) or brain damage, disorders of the heart or circulation.

An ECG should be done before treatment begins, due to reports of sudden unexplained death. This should be repeated after one year, when treatment must be reviewed and either stopped or reduced (under close supervision).

Regular monitoring of heart function should be done in those people receiving 16 mg daily or more. Patients receiving 6 mg daily or more should carry a treatment card indicating dosage.

Effects
General: drowsiness, weakness, temperature changes
Gastrointestinal: dry mouth, nausea, constipation, increased salivation
Urogenital: impotence
Central nervous system: tremor, rigidity, slow movement, physical restlessness, muscle spasms of neck, shoulders and trunk leading to abnormal postures, headache, EEG changes, convulsions, dizziness, vertigo
Endocrine: raised serum prolactin levels, breast enlargement in men
Women's health: scanty or no periods, secretion of milk from breasts
Psychological: insomnia, anxiety
Skin: rash, excessive sweating

Strength level: 4

Risperidone

Generic name	Brand name	Dosage
risperidone	Risperdal	2 mg daily (starting dose), increasing to 6–10 mg, sometimes up to 16 mg daily (maintenance dose)

Table 18.19: Risperidone

Uses: schizophrenia

Cautions: low blood pressure (particularly on standing), disorders of the heart or circulation (e.g. heart failure, heart attack, abnormal heart rhythms), dehydration or cerebrovascular disease, Parkinson's disease, epilepsy

Effects
General: allergic reactions, sleepiness, fatigue, disturbances in temperature regulation
Cardiovascular: low blood pressure, high blood pressure, palpitations, rapid heart rate, oedema
Respiratory: stuffy, runny nose
Gastrointestinal: constipation, indigestion, nausea, vomiting, abdominal pain, weight gain, increased salivation, raised liver enzymes
Urogenital: priapism, disturbances of penile erection and ejaculation, disorders of orgasm, incontinence
Central nervous system: headache, dizziness, impaired concentration, tremor, slow movements, physically restless, rigidity, dizziness on standing, tardive dyskinesia, neuroleptic malignant syndrome, convulsions, muscle spasms of neck, shoulders and trunk leading to abnormal postures
Endocrine: breast enlargement in men
Women's health: disturbances of the menstrual cycle, secretion of milk from breasts, cessation of periods
Psychological: anxiety, insomnia, agitation
Blood: low platelet count leading to bleeding into the skin, prolonged bleeding after injury and spontaneous bruising, *reduction of neutrophils* (type of white blood cell) leading to increased susceptibility to infection
Skin: rash
Special senses: blurred vision

Strength level: 4

Olanzapine

Generic name	Brand name	Dosage
olanzapine	Zyprexa	10–20 mg daily

Table 18.20: Olanzapine

Uses: schizophrenia

When not to be used: narrow-angle glaucoma

Cautions: enlarged prostate, paralytic ileus and related conditions, raised liver enzymes, signs and symptoms of liver impairment, use of drugs that affect the liver, low white blood cell counts, a history of drug-induced bone marrow depression or toxicity, increased eosinophils, bone marrow disease, a history of convulsions.

The blood pressure must be monitored regularly in patients over 65.

Effects
General: sleepiness
Cardiovascular: low blood pressure (particularly on standing), oedema in lower limbs
Gastrointestinal: weight gain, increased appetite, constipation, dry mouth, raised liver enzymes, hepatitis, raised blood sugar levels, destabilisation of diabetes mellitus
Urogenital: priapism
Musculoskeletal: high creatine phosphokinase
Central nervous system: dizziness, convulsions, neuroleptic malignant syndrome
Endocrine: breast enlargement in men, raised prolactin levels
Women's health: secretion of milk from breasts, breast enlargement
Blood: reduction in white blood cell count that may lead to increased infections, low *platelet count* leading to bleeding into the skin, prolonged bleeding after injury and spontaneous bruising
Skin: sensitivity to light, rash

Strength level: 4

Quetiapine

Generic name	Brand name	Dosage
quetiapine	Seroquel	300–450 mg daily

Table 18.21: Quetiapine

Uses: schizophrenia

Cautions: kidney impairment, the elderly, cerebrovascular disease

Effects
General: drowsiness, weakness, fever
Cardiovascular: palpitations, rapid heart rate, raised serum cholesterol and triglyceride levels
Respiratory: runny nose
Gastrointestinal: indigestion, constipation, dry mouth, raised liver enzymes
Musculoskeletal: muscle pain
Endocrine: reduced thyroid hormone levels
Psychological: anxiety
Blood: reduction in white blood cell count that may lead to increased infections, reduction of neutrophils (type of white blood cell) leading to increased susceptibility to infection, *increase in numbers of eosinophils* (type of white blood cell) usually denoting allergic reaction
Skin: rash

Strength level: 4

Sertindole

Generic name	Brand name	Dosage
sertindole	Serdolect, Serlect	12–24 mg daily

Table 18.22: Sertindole

Sertindole has been suspended following reports of arrhythmias and sudden cardiac death. It remains available on a named-patient basis (from Lundbeck) for patients already stabilised on the drug and in whom other antipsychotics are inappropriate. Because of the side-effects, 14% of patients had to stop taking the drug during clinical trials.

Strength level: 4

Ziprasidone

Generic name	Brand name	Dosage
ziprasidone	Geodon	20–160 mg daily

Table 18.23: Ziprasidone

Uses: schizophrenia

When not to be used: recent heart attack, heart failure.

Sudden unexplained deaths have occurred in people taking this drug. This can happen with all the 'major' tranquillisers but probably occurs most frequently with ziprasidone.

Cautions: disorders of the heart and circulation (e.g. history of heart attack, heart failure or abnormal heart rhythms), cerebrovascular disease, epilepsy or history of convulsions, situations leading to increases in temperature (e.g. strenuous exercise, hot environments), dehydration, drugs that cause dryness or heat (e.g. anticholinergics), the elderly, patients with confusion (there is a risk of aspiration pneumonia if swallowing is affected), low blood pressure or tendency to low blood pressure (e.g. dehydration or treatment with high blood pressure medication).

Serum potassium and magnesium levels should be determined before treatment in patients at risk of fluid or salt disturbances (e.g. diuretic use, diarrhoea or fluid loss). Low serum potassium or magnesium levels increase the risk of heart complications with this drug.

Symptoms of dizziness, palpitations or fainting need further investigation by 24-hour heart monitoring.

Rash or nettle rash is seen in about 5% of people treated and some of those have to stop treatment as a result. Some patients with rashes also have raised white blood cell counts and symptoms of systemic illness.

Effects (more than 4% of people given ziprasidone had to stop treatment because of side-effects)
> *General:* sleepiness, weakness, influenza-like symptoms, fever, decreased body temperature, accidental falls, chills, flank pain, back pain, road traffic accident, lymphatic gland enlargement
> *Cardiovascular:* low blood pressure (particularly on standing), ECG (EKG)

changes, palpitations, rapid heart rate, slow heart rate, high blood pressure, angina pectoris, abnormal heart rhythms that can be fatal, phlebitis, enlarged heart, deep vein thrombosis, inflammation of heart muscle, high blood pressure, vasodilatation, swelling of lower limbs, raised serum cholesterol levels, low serum cholesterol levels

Respiratory: swelling of the face, runny nose, cough, breathlessness, pneumonia, nosebleeds, coughing blood, stridor, pulmonary embolism

Gastrointestinal: nausea, constipation, indigestion, diarrhoea, dry mouth, poor appetite, increased salivation, weight gain, abdominal pain, vomiting, rectal bleeding, difficulty swallowing, swelling of the tongue, bleeding gums, jaundice, raised liver enzymes, vomiting blood, jaundice, hepatitis, enlargement of the liver, leucoplakia of mouth, bleeding from the bowel, thirst, low blood sugar levels, raised blood sugar levels, raised serum cholesterol levels, dehydration, rectal bleeding

Urogenital: impotence, abnormal ejaculation, blood in the urine, frequent urination, urinary retention, male sexual dysfunction, no orgasm, sugar in the urine, urination at night, scanty urination, priapism, protein in the urine, raised serum urea and creatinine levels, low serum protein levels

Musculoskeletal: muscle pain, joint pain, gout, tenosynovitis, weakness and wasting of muscles, raised serum uric acid levels, raised serum creatine phosphokinase (CPK) levels, low serum calcium and magnesium levels

Central nervous system: Parkinson's disease-like symptoms, physical restlessness, dizziness, muscle spasms of neck, shoulders and trunk leading to abnormal postures, increased muscle tone, tremor, involuntary and abnormal movements, pins and needles and numbness, vertigo, abnormal gait, spasmodic fixed deviation of eyes, increased sensitivity to touch, loss of balance, low muscle tone, lack of movement, difficulty speaking, tardive dyskinesia, lack of co-ordination, neuropathy, muscle spasms, pins and needles around the mouth, neck and back stiffness and muscle spasm, increased tendon reflexes, spasm of jaw muscles leading to inability to open mouth, headache, speech disorder, stroke, convulsions in 0.4% of patients

Endocrine: hypothyroidism, hyperthyroidism, inflammation of thyroid gland, breast enlargement in men, low blood sugar

Women's health: painful periods, no periods, heavy periods, flooding, secretion of breast milk, sexual disorders, vaginal bleeding

Psychological: agitation, personality disorder, psychosis, insomnia, anxiety, confusion, loss of memory, hostility

Blood: anaemia, increase in number of white blood cells, reduction in white blood cell count that may lead to increased infections, *increase in numbers of eosinophils* (type of white blood cell) usually denoting allergic reaction, *low platelet count* leading to bleeding into the skin, prolonged bleeding after injury and spontaneous bruising, increase in number of lymphocytes (type of white blood cell), increase in number of monocytes (type of white blood cell), increase in number of basophils (type of white blood cell), excess production of red blood cells due to bone marrow disturbance leading to thrombosis and bleeding, raised platelet levels due to bone marrow disturbance leading to thrombosis and bleeding, low potassium levels, low sodium levels, low or high chloride levels

Skin: rash, fungal skin infections, sensitivity to light, maculopapular rash, nettle rash, loss of head hair, eczema, exfoliative dermatitis (severe skin condition characterised by fever, redness, itching and scaling of skin), contact dermatitis, blistering rash, boils, sweating, bleeding into the skin

Special senses: abnormal vision, double vision, dry eyes, tinnitus, inflamed eyelids, cataract, sensitivity of eyes to light, eye haemorrhage, reduced field of vision, keratitis, conjunctivitis, rapid involuntary eye movements

Strength level: 4

Amisulpride

Generic name	Brand name	Dosage
amisulpride	Solian	400–800 mg daily (maximum 1.2 g daily)

Table 18.24: Amisulpride

Uses: schizophrenia

When not to be used: phaeochromocytoma, prolactin-dependent tumours

Cautions: kidney impairment, the elderly, those at risk of low blood pressure or sedation

Effects
General: drowsiness
Cardiovascular: low blood pressure, slow heart rate
Gastrointestinal: dry mouth, nausea, vomiting, constipation
Central nervous system: convulsions
Endocrine: raised serum prolactin levels, breast enlargement in men
Women's health: secretion of milk from breasts, no periods, breast pain, sexual dysfunction
Psychological: insomnia, anxiety, agitation

Strength level: 4

Zotepine

Generic name	Brand name	Dosage
zotepine	Zoleptil	25–100 mg 3 times daily

Table 18.25: Zotepine

Uses: schizophrenia

When not to be used: with high doses of other 'major' tranquillisers, gout (only to be given three weeks after attack subsides), history of kidney stones, sedation by other medications

Cautions: epilepsy or family history of epilepsy, liver or kidney impairment, enlarged prostate, urinary retention, narrow-angle glaucoma, paralytic ileus.

Because this drug leads to QT prolongation, as seen on ECG (EKG) recordings, an ECG must be performed before treatment begins.

Effects

General: weakness, drowsiness, fever, lowered body temperature

Cardiovascular: palpitations, rapid heart rate, slow heart rate, QT interval prolonged, high blood pressure, raised serum cholesterol levels, oedema

Respiratory: runny nose, flu-like symptoms, cough, breathlessness, nosebleeds

Gastrointestinal: poor appetite, thirst, nausea, vomiting, diarrhoea, constipation, indigestion, abdominal pain, dry mouth, raised liver enzymes, excess salivation, abdominal bloating, low blood sugar levels, high blood sugar levels

Urogenital: decreased libido, raised serum creatinine levels, impotence, incontinence, abnormal ejaculation, retention of urine

Musculoskeletal: low serum uric acid levels, muscle pain, joint pain, muscle weakness

Central nervous system: headache, EEG abnormalities, convulsions, speech disorder, vertigo, loss of balance, increased sensitivity to touch, muscle spasms

Endocrine: raised serum prolactin levels

Women's health: decreased libido, menstrual irregularities

Psychological: agitation, anxiety, depression, insomnia, confusion, loss of memory, coma

Blood: increase in number of white blood cells, reduction in white blood cell count that may lead to increased infections, *raised ESR, anaemia, excessive production of platelets* due to disturbance of marrow causing thrombosis and bleeding, *low platelet count* leading to bleeding into the skin, prolonged bleeding after injury and

spontaneous bruising
Skin: sweating, acne, dry skin, rash, loss of head hair, sensitivity to light
Special senses: blurred vision, conjunctivitis

Strength level: 4

Lithium

Technically, this drug is not a 'major' tranquilliser, but I have included it in this section as it is used for mental symptoms, in this case mania.

Generic name	Brand name	Dosage
lithium	Camcolit, Cibalith-S, Efalith*, Eskalith, Li-liquid, Liskonum, Litarex, Lithane, Lithobid, Lithonate, Lithotabs, Litharex, Phasal, Priadel	0.25 mg–2 g daily (dosage may vary according to individual response)

Table 18.26: Lithium

Uses: manic depression

When not to be used: kidney disease, cardiovascular disease, Addison's disease, heart failure, kidney impairment, untreated hypothyroidism

Cautions: regular monitoring is essential in all patients and there should be regular checks of kidney function, urine analysis, serum urea and creatinine, thyroid and heart function. All patients should be given information about the symptoms of lithium toxicity. They should be told to report excessive urination or thirst, nausea and vomiting and any other conditions that lead to dehydration. Elderly people are particularly liable to develop such symptoms and all patients should be regularly monitored.

Effects
Cardiovascular: oedema, palpitations, slow heart rate, abnormal heart rhythms, cardiomyopathy (enlarged heart, heart failure, palpitations, embolism), ECG changes
Gastrointestinal: thirst, nausea, weight gain
Urogenital: excessive urination
Musculoskeletal: muscle weakness, raised serum calcium and magnesium levels

Central nervous system: vertigo, hand tremors
Psychological: dazed feeling, amnesia
Endocrine: hyperparathyroidism, disturbances of thyroid function such as goitre, hypothyroidism and hyperthyroidism
Blood: increase in number of white blood cells
Skin: acne, psoriasis (including pustular psoriasis), rash, leg ulcers

Strength level: 4

CENTRAL NERVOUS SYSTEM STIMULANTS

Methylphenidate

Generic name	Brand name	Dosage
methylphenidate	Equasym, Ritalin	Children over 6 years: 5–40 mg daily

Table 18.27: Methylphenidate

Uses: attention deficit hyperactivity disorder (ADHD)

When not to be used: marked anxiety, agitation or tension, motor tics, tics in siblings, family history or diagnosis of Tourette's syndrome, hyperthyroidism, severe angina pectoris, abnormal heart rhythms, glaucoma, hyperthyroidism, children under six years of age, severe depression

Cautions: emotionally unstable patients. Ritalin should be used with caution in patients with epilepsy.

Treatment must only be given after obtaining a detailed history. A thorough assessment of the child's age and the severity of symptoms must be done before any decision is made to prescribe Ritalin.

Blood pressure, growth and development should be monitored regularly and thoroughly. Regular monitoring of blood counts is advisable.

Effects
General: drowsiness, fever, retarded growth and lack of weight gain in children
Cardiovascular: palpitations, rapid heart rate, abnormal heart rhythms, high blood pressure, low blood pressure, angina pectoris
Gastrointestinal: decreased appetite, abdominal pain, nausea, vomiting, dry mouth,

raised liver enzymes, liver coma

Musculoskeletal: muscle cramps, joint pains

Central nervous system: headache, dizziness, involuntary movements, convulsions, tics, exacerbation of existing tics, Tourette's syndrome, abnormal movements, cerebral arteritis and/or occlusion, neuroleptic malignant syndrome

Psychological: nervousness, hyperactivity, insomnia, depression, psychosis, hallucinations

Blood: reduction in white blood cell count that may lead to increased infections, *low platelet count* leading to bleeding into the skin, prolonged bleeding after injury and spontaneous bruising, *anaemia*

Skin: rash, itching, nettle rash, loss of head hair, skin inflammation with flaking and scaling, erythema multiforme

Special senses: difficulties in focusing, blurred vision

Strength level: 4

Notes

[1] *Beyond Prozac: Healing Mental Suffering Without Drugs* by Dr Terry Lynch (Mercier Press, 2001).

[2] Maprotiline, mianserin and trazodone are not, strictly speaking, tricyclic antidepressants but are included here as they have a similar side-effect profile.

[3] Also known as neuroleptics.

[4] For further information, see *www.nmsis.org.*

[5] There are also many sources of support for people and their families. These include Dr Peter Breggin (website: *www.breggin.com*) in the US, who is an outspoken critic of conventional psychiatric treatments.

19 STOMACH AND DUODENAL ULCER

There are many remedies for upper abdominal discomfort and pain that are available both over the counter and on prescription. These fall into two main groups: those used to neutralise acid and those that have anti-ulcer properties. The latter were originally given only in cases of proven peptic ulcers, but, in recent years (and increasingly), they are also given in cases where no ulcer is seen on investigation or even without any investigation performed.

This use of powerful drugs for simple indigestion is often inappropriate and presents problems for patients and for holistic practitioners. They are powerful suppressive agents. When the drugs are given, they very quickly relieve the symptoms of peptic ulceration or indigestion. However, when they are stopped, a rebound appearance of the same symptoms can occur, even after several years. It has been recognised for a long time that maintenance therapy is often necessary, when a reduced dosage is taken at night. Even if the drug was originally used for gastrointestinal haemorrhage, there may be a recurrence when the drug is finally stopped. There is some evidence that long-term use of these drugs may actually lead to the development of gastric carcinoma. It is known that this condition is related to low or absent gastric acid. These drugs produce such a state.

PROTON PUMP INHIBITORS

Generic name	Brand name	Dosage
esomeprazole	Nexium	20–40 mg daily
lansoprazole	Zoton	15–30 mg daily
omeprazole	Losec, Prilosec	10–40 mg daily (maximum 120 mg daily)
pantoprazole	Protium	40 mg daily
rabeprazole	Pariet	20 mg daily

Table 19.1: Proton pump inhibitors

Uses: stomach and duodenal ulcer, indigestion, heartburn

Cautions: liver disease, the diagnosis of stomach cancer may be delayed because this drug hides its symptoms

Effects

Cardiovascular: oedema
Respiratory: wheezing, swelling of face and upper body
Gastrointestinal: diarrhoea, constipation, nausea, vomiting, flatulence, abdominal pain, dry mouth, sore mouth, oral thrush, taste disturbance, hepatitis, jaundice, liver failure, raised liver enzymes
Urogenital: nephritis, kidney impairment, impotence
Musculoskeletal: joint pain, muscle pain
Central nervous system: dizziness, headache, pins and needles, vertigo
Endocrine: breast enlargement in men
Psychological: confusion, sleepiness, insomnia, confusion, agitation, depression, hallucinations
Blood: reduction in white blood cell count that may lead to increased infections, *low platelet count* leading to bleeding into the skin, prolonged bleeding after injury and spontaneous bruising, *severe acute reduction in numbers of neutrophils* (type of white blood cell) leading to severe bacterial infections that are usually fatal, *reduction in numbers of red and white blood cells and platelets* leading to anaemia, increased risk of infection and spontaneous bruising/bleeding
Skin: sweating, rash, nettle rash, itching, sensitivity to light, erythema multiforme, Stevens-Johnson syndrome (fever, blistering of mouth, throat, anus and eyes), toxic epidermal necrolysis (life-threatening condition where the skin peels off in sheets leaving areas stripped of skin), hair loss, large blisters

Strength level: 2

H₂ BLOCKERS

Generic name	Brand name	Dosage
cimetidine	Acitak, Algitec*, Cimagen, Cimeldine, Dyspamet, Galenamet, Peptimax, Phimetin, Tagamet, Tagamet Dual Action*, Ultec, Zita	800–2,400 mg daily
famotidine	Pepcid	20–40 mg twice daily
nizatidine	Axid	150–300 mg twice daily
ranitidine	Pylorid, Xanomel, Zandine, Zantac	150 mg–6g daily (depending on the condition being treated)

Table 19.2: H₂ blockers

Uses: stomach and duodenal ulcer, indigestion, heartburn

Cautions: the diagnosis of stomach cancer may be delayed because this drug hides its symptoms

Effects

General: tiredness, fever, severe allergic reaction

Cardiovascular: palpitations, vasculitis (inflammation of small blood vessels that may lead to skin rashes, arthritis, bruising of the skin and kidney failure)

Gastrointestinal: diarrhoea, raised liver enzymes, pancreatitis, poor appetite, dry mouth

Urogenital: nephritis, impotence, raised serum creatinine, kidney failure

Musculoskeletal: joint pain, muscle pain, arthritis

Central nervous system: dizziness, headache

Endocrine: breast enlargement in men

Psychological: confusion, mood and behavioural changes, insomnia, depression, hallucinations, anxiety

Blood: low platelet count leading to bleeding into the skin, prolonged bleeding after injury and spontaneous bruising, *reduction in white blood cell count* that may lead to increased infections, *severe acute reduction in numbers of neutrophils* (type of white blood cell) leading to severe bacterial infections that are usually fatal, *reduction in numbers of red and white blood cells and platelets* leading to anaemia, increased risk of infection and spontaneous bruising/bleeding

Skin: bruising of the skin, rash, hair loss, toxic epidermal necrolysis (life-threatening condition where the skin peels off in sheets leaving areas stripped of skin), nettle rash

Strength level: 2

CARBENOXOLONE

Generic name	Brand name	Dosage
carbenoxolone	Bioplex, Bioral, Pyrogastrone*	100 mg daily (by mouth)

Table 19.3: Carbenoxolone

Uses: inflammation and ulceration of oesophagus

When not to be used: low potassium levels, heart failure, those receiving digoxin (unless electrolyte levels are checked every week)

Cautions: heart disease, high blood pressure, liver and kidney impairment, the elderly

Effects
>*General:* low potassium levels
>*Cardiovascular:* high blood pressure, heart failure

Strength level: 2

MISOPROSTOL

Generic name	Brand name	Dosage
misoprostol	Arthrotec*, Cytotec, Napratec*	400–800 mcg daily

Table 19.4: Misoprostol

Uses: stomach or duodenal ulcers

When not to be used: obstructive disorders of the digestive system, kidney failure, with oral antibiotics such as erythromycin, clarithromycin or troleandomycin or with antiviral agent nefazodone

Cautions: liver or kidney impairment or renal insufficiency, chronic lung disease, respiratory failure, history of heart disease, Parkinson's disease, Parkinson's disease-like symptoms

Effects
>*Cardiovascular:* palpitations, abnormal heart rhythms (which have caused deaths)
>*Respiratory:* wheezing, swelling of face and upper body
>*Gastrointestinal:* abdominal cramps, diarrhoea, borborygmi, raised liver enzymes
>*Urogenital:* frequent urination
>*Central nervous system:* headache, light-headedness, convulsions, Parkinson's disease-like symptoms
>*Endocrine:* raised serum prolactin levels, breast enlargement in men
>*Women's health:* secretion of milk from breasts
>*Skin:* rash, itching, nettle rash

Strength level: 2

HOLISTIC MANAGEMENT

When dealing with upper abdominal problems such as indigestion or even peptic ulcer, remember that antacids are used for symptomatic relief. Reduction of anti-ulcer drugs can lead to reappearance of the original symptom picture and must be done slowly, in conjunction with holistic treatment. The antacid can be dealt with subsequently. Frequent use of antacids actually leads to secretion of *increased* levels of acid as the stomach tries to maintain a normal level of pH. If reduction of the antacid is too rapid, then the upper gastrointestinal tract will be exposed to the full force of this increased acid level.

The removal of other factors that tend to lead to increases in acid, such as cigarettes, coffee, acid foods and spices, will all help in this process. Bowel disorders in general often respond well to holistic medical treatment and, once the more powerful anti-ulcer drugs have been removed, progress should be more rapid.

20 DRUGS NECESSARY FOR LIFE

Drugs that are necessary to maintain life are categorised as Level 5 on page 22. It is an extreme of drug use, but is not as common as one would first suppose. If a patient does take these drugs, it is important that you seek advice and help from a conventionally trained medical practitioner.

HEART DRUGS

Drugs may be used in severe and serious abnormalities of heart rhythm. Anatomically, such abnormalities arise from the ventricle and are diagnosed clinically, but the precise differentiation is by means of an ECG. The main symptom is palpitations.

Such drugs are not commonly encountered and are listed on page 23. If any of these drugs are seen, their dosage must not be altered without close liaison with a conventionally trained doctor, as any inappropriate reduction in dosage may lead to a fatal cardiac arrhythmia.

Betablockers may be given to prevent or treat abnormal heart rhythms, so it is important to check their indication in each case. They are generally given for abnormal rhythms arising from the atrium, not the ventricle, and therefore are not life-threatening. Betablockers can be dealt with as outlined on page 123.

ENDOCRINE DISEASE

In endocrine disease, there is overactivity or underactivity of an endocrine gland due to a disease process. Women who are given oestrogen during or after the menopause (which is not a disease) or who take the contraceptive pill do not come into this category. The use of female sex hormones is described on page 89.

DIABETES MELLITUS

A differentiation must be made between insulin-dependent and non-insulin-dependent types of diabetes mellitus. The difficulty is that diabetes mellitus that is treated by either insulin or hypoglycaemic agents may be complicated by the development of hypoglycaemia – 'hypos'. This may manifest merely as hunger or light-headedness. Coma may develop when the blood sugar falls to very low levels, as can happen in insulin-dependent diabetes. Death can occur if the blood sugar level continues to fall.

The risk of low blood sugar levels developing must be minimised as much as possible. In the case of patients who take insulin, this acts rapidly and the dosage and adjustment of dosage is complex, so regular monitoring is important. It may be preferable for a medical practitioner to supervise such cases.

During holistic treatment, the blood sugar should be monitored frequently every day. The blood sugar is likely to fall with treatment as pancreatic function improves and blood sugar levels stabilise. The insulin dosage needs to be adjusted in response to this. This will be a continuous process as, hopefully, the condition improves.

It is unusual for people to be able to stop their insulin completely, but either the dose can be reduced or cases of 'brittle' or unstable diabetes can be stabilised. In both cases, such patients feel better in themselves with more energy.

In non-insulin-dependent diabetes mellitus, most cases are relatively simple to manage. Again, the problem with the hypoglycaemic agents is that they can induce hypoglycaemia. With due care, it is possible to begin a strict diet and reduce drug dosage according to blood sugar levels whilst treating. Monitoring of the blood sugar will ensure that very high levels of blood sugar are not attained.

The patient may also take steps to ensure that their activities do not lead to raised blood sugar. They should avoid stressful situations, smoking and taking coffee or stimulant drugs. As treatment progresses, the blood sugar level should fall as the patient's condition improves. Do not worry if the patient only feels better initially with improved energy levels but little change in the blood sugar. Falls in sugar level follow these improvements.

Symptoms and signs to be concerned about in either type of diabetes are a rising blood sugar level, deterioration in feeling of wellness, the appearance of ketones in the urine and worsening of symptoms such as frequency and volume of urination, thirst and appetite and occurrence of hypoglycaemic episodes. In these cases, either more frequent treatment is necessary, a review of treatment is required or conventional medical treatment may need to be instituted in extreme situations.

THYROID DISEASE

Thyroid hormone replacement therapy

Thyroid hormone replacement therapy (thyroxine) is used in cases of hypothyroidism – underactivity of thyroid gland function. The disease tends to be variable in its manifestations and there may be a progressive element. Annual checks of thyroid hormone levels are advised in conventional medicine. Holistic treatment can improve thyroid function, so checking of thyroid hormone levels should be done more frequently. I arrange for blood levels to be checked every three or six months, with reversion to annual checks after treatment has ended. If necessary, the dosage of thyroid replacement is altered in accordance with the blood level.

Anti-thyroid drugs

Anti-thyroid drugs such as carbimazole and methimazole are used in the treatment of hyperthyroidism. When dealing with patients who take such medication, it is important to bear in mind that this can be a serious condition. Management must include estimation of serum thyroxine levels.

Most patients tend to decide on conventional treatment when first diagnosed and so present for holistic treatment later. Reduction of these drugs can only take place as levels of thyroxine in the blood fall.

Routine conventional management of the condition is for the patient to take the drug for a year or so. Effective holistic treatment may well reduce this period and end with an improved state of health. As with many conditions, it is clearly more beneficial if patients present for treatment as soon as they notice symptoms (if not before). Any delay, as often occurs when conventional investigations are undertaken, will make it more difficult to treat such patients.

In my experience of treating overactive thyroid disease, people respond well to holistic treatment. There is frequently a preceding emotional shock or upset before the onset of the symptoms and it is helpful to address this, perhaps with counselling or relaxation and meditation. Such support, in addition to holistic treatment, is very beneficial in dealing with the underlying imbalances responsible for thyroid disease.

DIABETES INSIPIDUS

In cases of diabetes insipidus, the vasopressin (antidiuretic hormone) is never stopped and people must be treated in liaison with a conventionally trained doctor.

ADDISON'S DISEASE (INSUFFICIENCY OF ADRENAL CORTEX)

Patients with Addison's disease take a mixture of corticosteroids, a glucocorticoid such as cortisone or prednisolone and a mineralocorticoid (fludrocortisone). These drugs must not be altered or stopped at all and monitoring must be performed in conjunction with conventional medical advice.

Do not confuse the use of these drugs for Addison's disease and when given for their anti-inflammatory effect in disorders such as rheumatoid arthritis, ulcerative colitis, asthma and so on. Cortisone and hydrocortisone have mixed glucocorticoid/ mineralocorticoid actions and so may be prescribed in inflammatory disease. Fludrocortisone is only ever used in cases of insufficiency of the adrenal cortex.

21 ENERGETIC VIEW OF PRESCRIBED DRUGS

Chinese medicine provides a model of subtle energetic anatomy and physiology that can give insights into drug actions. One difficulty in treating patients is to predict what may happen when they take drugs. With an understanding of the principles of Chinese medicine, it is possible to interpret the actions of prescribed drugs. This helps us understand how drugs affect us and how best to mitigate the worst of their harmful actions.

The best method of determining the actions of drugs is for practitioners to take them themselves. Traditionally, practitioners would determine the energetic actions of herbs by testing them personally. Over many years of observation, it was possible to study their effects. In this way, some became part of the Chinese herbal medicine pharmacopoeia and others were rejected.

Homoeopaths test substances in a similar way with 'provings'. Healthy volunteers are given a substance and they record any and all symptoms that are produced. This is a thoroughly scientific and reproducible method of determining the actions of a substance. Information can also be gathered from studies of toxicology, clinical trials and from clinical observations.

Therefore, we can begin to understand how prescribed drugs affect the body, its organs, the Qi and Blood. Such information is very valuable, because practitioners can tailor treatment to take account of such effects and can also give patients information about the effects of drugs.

The study of Chinese herbs can lead us to draw some conclusions about prescribed medication. Chinese herbs are categorised according to their main action – clearing Heat, tonifying Qi and so forth. This includes information about:

- direction of action (ascending or descending);
- Qi (warm, cold, hot or cool);
- taste (sweet, salty, bland, sour, acrid, aromatic, bitter): and
- organs affected.

There is some value in trying to determine the qualities of Western medications in the same way. There is a lot of work to be done in this area and this is, by no means, a definitive account.[1] This process is still in its early stages. It is also not necessary to analyse medications as deeply or profoundly as the Chinese medical community have done with herbs over generations, as the intention is not to use the drugs in treatment. The main intention here is to facilitate the patient in reducing medication, when appropriate, so that their health can be maximised both from holistic treatment and from the removal of disease-producing chemicals.

I find it useful in my own practice to analyse the effects of drugs, as it makes treatment much more simple. If we know the energetic effects of drugs, we can adjust treatment principles more accurately to take account of them.

One way of looking at Western medications is to see if there are any that are derived from herbal sources. A good example is ephedrine, which is derived from Ma Huang *Herba Ephedrae*. Some similarities can therefore be deduced from a study of this herb. Ma Huang *Herba Ephedrae* is a warm, acrid and bitter herb that releases the Exterior, disperses Cold, stops wheezing, softens the Lungs and has diuretic actions.

The Western drug ephedrine has similar actions in inducing sweating (by releasing the Exterior) and relieving wheezing. It is not much used nowadays, but several drugs have ephedrine-like actions. These include the beta-adrenoceptor stimulant bronchodilators described on page 65. We can now understand the consequences of prolonged bronchodilator use: Lung Qi Deficiency, due to continued dispersion of Lung Qi; Heat in the Lung or Lung Yin Deficiency, due to their warming actions and their ability to produce sweating; as well as Heart Qi Deficiency, as the drug damages Heart Qi and circulation.

Another way of determining the action of a drug is to consider the effect it is trying to produce. For example, Valium is used as a sedative, a tranquilliser and to induce sleep. In an excellent article in his book *Something Old, Something New*,[2] Bob Flaws desribes the energetic effects of Valium as having an effect on Calming the Spirit. This category of Chinese herbs is used to treat symptoms such as irritability and insomnia. They act mainly by virtue of their weight and density as they settle and calm the Spirit. They are used to treat Heart symptoms such as palpitations, anxiety and insomnia and Liver symptoms such as dizziness and irritability. They easily injure Stomach Qi, leading to indigestion and loss of appetite. They are invariably used together with herbs that nourish and strengthen Spleen and Stomach Qi. The drugs that are classified as 'major' tranquillisers also have a strong effect on Calming the Spirit.

Non-steroidal anti-inflammatory drugs are intended to treat the pain and joint swelling of arthritis as well as musculoskeletal pain in general and dysmenorrhoea.

Similar actions are produced by a category of Chinese herbs that Disperse Wind Damp – most are used for Wind Damp Cold conditions and some for Wind Damp Heat conditions. They are generally acrid in nature and are used to treat Bi syndrome by dispersing Wind Dampness from the muscles, sinews, joints and bones. Therefore, long-term use of such herbs (and medications such as NSAIDs) leads to Qi Deficiency (due to their dispersing action), Yin and Blood Deficiency (which is why regular prescription of NSAIDs leads to more joint problems and eventually kidney disease) and Heat in the Stomach.

Other medications may be less easy to compare with herbal categories, although they have powerful effects on health. For example, betablockers produce effects such as cold extremities, slow pulse, tiredness, impotence, wheezing and low blood pressure. They are cold in nature and mainly affect the Liver, Kidney, Spleen, Heart and Lungs. If a patient who is constitutionally cold takes them, they will experience such symptoms very quickly and find that the drugs make them quite ill. However, if a patient who is constitutionally hot takes them, the side-effects (at least in the short term) will be much milder.

Female sex hormones produce symptoms of Qi and eventually Blood Stagnation. They do this because they are cold in nature and cause sluggishness and slowing of Qi flow. Their effects will be much stronger and more unpleasant in women who are Yang and Qi Deficient. Those who are Yin Deficient with Excess Yang will often feel subjectively better. Of course, long-term use of cold drugs will deplete anyone and therefore lead to difficulties later. Long-term use of female sex hormones is connected to Blood Stagnation syndromes such as cancer.

An important point to consider in determing the appropriate treatment is the concept in Chinese medicine of *Ben* and *Biao*, root and branch. *Ben* and *Biao* allow us to determine what to treat first – what are our priorities. There are almost always both aspects to consider in any patient. The root, or *Ben*, is to do with underlying imbalances (the origin of chronic disease), while the manifestation, *Biao*, is the subsequent problem, the manifesting symptoms and a more acute situation. It is essential to determine what is the relative importance of these two principles. However, they are not separate but are interconnected, as all symptoms are connected to underlying energetic imbalances.

This is why conventional drug medication leads to further health problems, as they only treat the manifestation, *Biao*, and take no account of the root, *Ben*. For example, high blood pressure due to Liver Yang Rising resulting from Kidney Yin Deficiency is a common scenario. The branch, *Biao*, of Liver Yang Rising needs to be considered along with the root, *Ben*, of Kidney Yin Deficiency. Effective treatment has to be directed at both aspects. Prescribed drug treatment is only ever directed at the branch, *Biao*. It cannot and does not address the root, *Ben*, since conventional medicine has no philosophical basis with which to determine underlying energetic imbalances. So, although treating the manifestion (*Biao*) can and does lead to removal of symptoms, as in the treatment of hypertension by drugs, long-term the root (*Ben*) can only be made worse.

Another way of explaining this is that the body adjusts to the external influence of the drugs yet is not balanced in any healthy way. When the drugs are stopped, symptoms return, usually stronger than before, and the underlying root (*Ben*) has usually been made worse. Whilst people are taking the drugs, they have two problems: the original energetic imbalance and the negative effects of the drugs. When people stop or reduce medication, they suffer withdrawal symptoms as the suppressed branch (*Biao*) flares up.

The key, as always, is to take the case, make a diagnosis and decide upon treatment principles. The treatment principles may need to be adjusted to reflect the use of prescribed drugs (as, indeed, they would be amended for any lifestyle activity, such as drinking alcohol, excessive exercise and so forth). Once the practitioner has decided on the appropriate treatment principles, treatment can begin. This can be amended during the course of treatment, depending on the patient's responses to treatment and, if appropriate, any drug reduction.

The information listed in Table 21.1 is an analysis of the common drugs used in conventional medicine in terms of their energetic effects.

Prescribed drug	Conventional use	Chinese medicine – analysis of effects	Treatment principle for ameliorating effects[3]
ACE inhibitors	Hypertension, heart failure	Blood Heat	Cool Blood
		Stomach Heat	Cool Stomach
		Heat in the Liver	Cool Liver
		Lung Yin Deficiency	Tonify Lung Yin
Antibiotics (excluding sulphonamides)	Bacterial infection	Spleen Qi Deficiency	Tonify Spleen Qi
		Blood Heat	Cool Blood
		Blood Deficiency	Tonify Blood
		Damp Accumulation	Drain or transform Damp

Antidepressants	Depression, enuresis in children	Liver Wind	Calm Liver Wind
		Blood and Spleen Qi Deficiency	Tonify Blood and Spleen Qi
		Heat in the Liver	Cool Liver
		Heart Qi Deficiency	Tonify Heart Qi
		Stomach Heat	Cool Stomach
		Stomach Qi Rebelling Upwards	Subdue Rebellious Stomach Qi
Antifungal agents	Fungal infection	Blood Deficiency	Tonify Blood
		Stomach Qi Rebelling Upwards	Subdue Rebellious Stomach Qi
		Spleen Qi Deficiency	Tonify Spleen Qi
Antihistamines	Allergies such as hay fever and urticaria, insomnia in children	Heat in the Liver	Cool Liver
		Stomach Heat	Cool Stomach
		Stomach Qi Rebelling Upwards	Subdue Rebellious Stomach Qi
		Blood Deficiency	Tonify Blood
Aspirin and non-steroidal anti-inflammatory drugs	Pain, fever, arthritis	Stomach Qi Rebelling	Subdue Rebellious Stomach Qi
		Blood Deficiency	Tonify Blood
		Blood Heat	Cool Blood
		Heat in the Liver	Cool Liver
		Warm, acrid releasing the exterior	Tonify Lung Qi and Yin
Beta-adrenoceptor stimulant	Asthma, premature labour	Heat in Lung	Cool Lung
		Heat in Liver	Cool Liver
		Lung Qi and Yin Deficiency	Tonify Lung Qi and Yin
		Heart Qi Deficiency	Tonify Heart Qi

Betablocker	Hypertension, anxiety, hyperthyroidism, angina pectoris, migraine, palpitations	Deficiency of Qi and Yang – Spleen, Heart, Lung and Kidney	Tonify Qi and Yang
Calcium channel lockers	Hypertension, angina pectoris	Heat in Liver	Cool Liver
		Blood Heat	Cool Blood
		Heat in Stomach	Cool Stomach
		Qi Deficiency (Spleen)	Tonify Qi (Spleen)
Cholesterol-lowering drugs	High cholesterol levels	Heat in Stomach	Cool Stomach
		Heat in Liver	Cool Liver
Corticosteroids	Autoimmune disease, asthma, rheumatoid arthritis, Addison's disease, eczema and psoriasis, inflammatory bowel disease	Stomach Heat	Cool Stomach
		Deficiency of Blood, Spleen and Lung Qi	Tonify Blood, Spleen and Lung Qi
		DampHeat Accumulation	Clear Heat and Drain Damp
		Heart Heat	Cool Heart
		Disperse Lung Qi	Tonify Lung Qi and Yin, regulate water passages
Diuretics	Oedema, heart failure, hypertension	Stomach Qi Rebelling Upwards	Subdue Rebellious Stomach Qi
		Qi and Yin Deficiency	Tonify Qi and Blood
H$_2$ blockers	Indigestion, peptic ulcer	Stomach Qi Rebelling Upwards	Subdue Rebellious Stomach Qi
		Deficiency of Blood, Kidney and Qi (Spleen)	Tonify Blood, Kidney and Qi (Spleen)

Levodopa	Parkinson's disease	Heart Heat	Cool Heart
		Blood Heat	Cool Blood
		Blood Deficiency	Tonify Blood
		Liver Heat and Wind	Cool and calm Liver
		Stomach Qi Rebelling Upwards	Subdue Rebellious Stomach Qi
Major tranquillisers	Schizophrenia, delusional states	Stomach Heat	Cool Stomach
		Stomach Qi Rebelling Upwards	Subdue Rebellious Stomach Qi
		Qi Deficiency	Tonify Qi
		Liver Heat and Wind	Cool and calm Liver
		Heart Qi Deficiency	Tonify Heart Qi
		Blood Deficiency	Tonify Blood
Methotrexate, azathioprine	Autoimmune disease	Liver Heat	Cool Liver
		Heart Heat	Cool Heart
		Blood Heat	Cool Blood
		Blood Deficiency	Tonify Blood
		Heat in Stomach	Cool Stomach
Minor tranquillisers	Anxiety, insomnia	Stomach Qi Rebelling Upwards	Subdue Rebellious Stomach Qi
		Deficiency of Qi and Blood	Tonify Qi and Blood
		Stomach Heat	Cool Stomach
		Heart Qi Deficiency	Tonify Heart Qi
Nitrates	Angina pectoris, heart failure	Stomach Qi Rebelling Upwards	Subdue Rebellious Stomach Qi
		Heat in Liver	Cool Liver
		Heat in Heart	Cool Heart

Opiate pain reliever	Pain, diarrhoea	Lung Heat	Cool Lung
		Heart Heat	Cool Heart
		Stomach Qi Rebelling Upwards	Subdue Rebellious Stomach Qi
		Blood Heat	Cool Blood
		Liver Heat	Cool Liver
Paracetamol	Pain	Liver Heat	Cool Liver
Progesterone	As oestrogen	As oestrogen, with less cooling and stagnation syndromes	
Sodium valproate	Epilepsy	Stomach Heat	Cool Stomach
		Blood Deficiency	Tonify Blood
		Liver Heat	Cool Liver
		Heart Heat	Cool Heart
Sulphonamide antibacterial	Bacterial infection	Blood Heat	Cool Blood
		Blood Deficiency	Tonify Blood
		Stomach Qi Rebelling Upwards	Subdue Rebellious Stomach Qi
		Lung Yin Deficiency	Tonify Lung Yin
		Heat in Liver	Cool Liver
		DampHeat in Large Intestine	Regulate Large Intestine, clear Heat and Dampness

Table 21.1: Energetic effects of prescribed drugs

HERB–DRUG INTERACTIONS

There is a lot of discussion now about how herbs and drugs interact and possibly affect each other's actions. In the modern world, people have many choices available to them. One result is that many people take herbs and prescribed drugs at the same time. Currently, 18.4% of Americans (15 million) use herbs and drugs concurrently. This is an important area and it is helpful for herbalists, of whatever tradition, to be clear about how herbal treatment may need to be amended to take account of any prescribed drugs that the patient is taking.

A further complication is that there is an agenda amongst some members of the medical profession to use fears of herb–drug interactions as a way of restricting the use of herbal treatments. For example, when there are reports of a Chinese herb causing kidney damage, the medical press describes it as 'Chinese herb nephropathy', rather than using the name of the particular herb or contaminant in question. The implication is that all herbs are assumed to be responsible for causing problems. In conventional medicine, no one would dream of using the term 'prescribed drug nephropathy' when aspirin causes kidney disease. It is named 'analgesic nephropathy'. There are very few studies that present information about herb–drug interactions and there is a consequent lack of information in this area. In addition, even when there are reports of interactions or problems, it is difficult to discover the provenance of some of these reports.

There are two difficulties that may arise when people take herbs together with drugs: either the effects of the drugs are increased or they are decreased. Regarding pharmacology and the chemical actions of drugs, there may be interactions between substances due to changes in absorption, distribution, metabolism or elimination. Many of the theoretical conclusions about herb–drug interactions come from analyses on how herbs affect these functions within the body. There has been some published material, but, in many cases, their conclusions are based on these theoretical ideas rather than clinical experience. For example, some laxatives are thought to cause problems with digoxin because fluid and potassium loss may lead to increased digoxin sensitivity.

I find that clinical experience is by far the most effective method of gathering information. From the perspective of Chinese medicine, it is helpful to assess the *energetic* actions of drugs (see Table 21.1), as this will lead to an effective therapeutic response based on an energetic analysis of the case. Careful observation of the patient is *the* method, *par excellence,* of determining the correct course of action. However, there is much work remaining to be done in this area and the pooling of clinical information amongst practitioners is very important. The Register of Chinese Herbal Medicine[4] in the UK is doing important work in this area, as is the Register of Medical Herbalists,[5] who work with herbs in the Western tradition. Further help can be requested from your local pharmacist, who has access to the latest information. Also, check out my website on *www.drgascoigne.com.*

Often, there is reticence on the part of patients about telling their doctor or health-care practitioner of other treatments they are taking. This is partly due to a fear of how their doctor will react to them taking herbal medicines. However, this needs to be overcome if people are to receive the best treatment possible. At least one practitioner needs to know everything that a patient is taking, so that an appropriate overall management plan can be determined. In my own practice, I find that patients are very open about their medications, herbs, vitamin and mineral supplements and so on. I discuss these with patients so that they can decide how to deal with them appropriately.

In my experience with Chinese medicine, it is not so much the individual herb that needs to be considered but the overall effect of the formula that is being used. For example, is the intention to tonify the Qi, move Blood, cool Heat and so on? Single herbs are not generally used in the Chinese tradition and, if they are, you need to be much more careful about their possible effects and their possible interactions with prescribed drugs. Generally, it is the complete herbal formula that needs to be considered, its overall function as well as the individual herbs it contains.

Firstly, problems may occur when the actions of the *formula* mimic the actions of the drugs. Dang Gui (*Radix Angelicae Sinensis*) is cited as interfering with Warfarin treatment to cause bleeding, because this herb has an action in moving the blood. However, this does not mean that Dang Gui *Radix Angelicae Sinensis* can never be used in patients taking Warfarin. I treat several patients who take Warfarin and I give virtually all of them Dang Gui *Radix Angelicae Sinensis* as only one herb of several in a formula. As Warfarin is heating and moving to the Blood, I use formulae that have some elements of cooling and nourishing the Blood. Dang Gui *Radix Angelicae Sinensis* may well be part of such a formula. Generally, I find that, as treatment continues, the regular blood tests that are done to check on the effectiveness of the Warfarin treatment settle down and the Warfarin dosage stabilises. Similarly, a strongly diuretic formula that Drains Damp would not be given if the patient is also taking prescribed diuretics.

The information in Table 21.1 regarding the energetic actions of drugs leads quite naturally to treatment principles that can be applied to moderate the drug's side-effects. For example, if a patient is taking antidepressants that create a lot of Heat in the Liver and Heart, treatment may need to be modified to cool the Heart and Liver somewhat. If the drug treatment has been more long term, it may well be necessary to pay attention to nourishing Heart and Liver Yin, as the effects of heat over a long period deplete the Yin. Eventually, Kidney Yin will be affected, of course. It is important to avoid a situation where a patient is, for example, taking antidepressants and a formula is also given that leads to heat in the Heart or Liver. This would only worsen any side-effects and make the patient feel more uncomfortable. Similarly, if a patient with asthma were taking bronchodilator medication, it would be wise to moderate the dosage of herbs that have a similar effect. Ma Huang *Herba Ephedrae* is the main herb to be circumspect about in such situations.

Of course, if patients are already taking bronchodilator medication, it may not be necessary to use many herbs to stop wheezing, in which case the underlying imbalance can be the main focus. This is the approach used by Giovanni Maciocia in the formulation of his herbal formulae for supporting patients who are receiving chemotherapy or radiotherapy. In *The Three Treasures News* of Autumn 1999, he outlines the effects of chemotherapy agents and how his formula, Chemo-support, can ameliorate the side-effects of such strong medication. It is not necessary to focus so much on the cancer, as the drugs are treating that. Similar comments can be made about the use of hormone replacement therapy at the menopause. The underlying imbalances can be focused on without needing to treat symptoms such as hot flushing and sweating.

One concern that is frequently expressed is that the use of herbs leads to *decreased* effectiveness of drugs. As I discussed in the Introduction (page 5), drugs are not intended to 'cure' but merely to remove symptoms. Herbal treatments, on the other hand, are used with the intention of remedying any underlying imbalance that may have led to the symptom in the first place. These are quite different processes, with quite different outcomes. The correct herbal treatment will lead to increased health, vitality and resistance to disease. Drugs erode our health and, although they may be necessary for life in a small proportion of cases (see Level 5 on page 22), they frequently lead to decreased vitality and lowered resistance to disease. The use of a correctly applied herbal treatment, therefore, can only lead to increased health, whatever drugs people are taking. I encourage patients and practitioners to use herbs, as the outcome can only be beneficial to the patient. It is sensible advice, however, to recommend that people take herbs and drugs separately (up to 3–4 hours apart) to prevent problems based on changes to the digestive system that can take place after medication is taken.

Notes

[1] Several authors and practitioners of Chinese medicine have written about the energetics of Western medication. These include: Bob Flaws, Blue Poppy Enterprises, 5441 Western Ave, #2, Boulder, CO 80301, USA (website: <http://www.bluepoppy.com>); Giovanni Maciocia, acupuncturist, medical herbalist and author of textbooks on Chinese medicine; Subhuti Dharmananda, Director of the Institute for Traditional Medicine, 2017 SE Hawthorne Blvd., Portland, OR 97214, USA (website: <http://www.itmonline.org>) John K. Chen, a specialist in pharmacy and traditional Chinese medicine; and Michael Tierra at the East West School of Herbology, P.O. Box 275, Ben Lomond, CA 95005, USA (website: <http://www.planetherbs.com>).

[2] *Something Old, Something New* by Bob Flaws (Blue Poppy Press, 1988).

[3] In this section, the precise treatment principle depends upon the situation. For example, although cholesterol-lowering drugs cause Heat in the Liver, it may be necessary to regulate Liver Qi, clear Liver Heat or tonify Liver Yin, depending on the person. Therefore, any mention in this column of cooling implies any of these specific treatment principles that are appropriate to the situation.

[4] Register of Chinese Herbal Medicine, Office 5, Ferndale Business Centre, 1 Exeter Street, Norwich NR2 4QB, UK. Email: *herbmed@rchm.com*. Website: *www.rchm.co.uk*.

[5] National Institute of Medical Herbalists, 56 Longbrook Street, Exeter, Devon EX4 6AH, UK. Email: *nimh@ukexeter.freeserve.co.uk*. Website: *www.nimh.org.uk*.

BIBLIOGRAPHY

Books

New Guide to Medicines and Drugs by John A. Henry (Dorling and Kindersley, 2000).
The British Medical Association's Concise Guide to Medicines and Drugs by John A. Henry (Dorling and Kindersley, 2001).
British National Formulary (BMJ Books, 2002). This is updated twice yearly in March and September and is widely used by medical practitioners. It is a clearly written guide to prescribed drugs. It has a limited amount of information about side-effects.
Martindale: The Complete Drug Reference edited by Sean Sweetman (Pharmaceutical Press, 2002).
Meyler's Side Effects of Drugs edited by M.N.G. Dukes (Elesevier, 1996).
ABPI Data Sheet Compendium. This is an annual publication that is a useful source of information for the medical profession (provided by the pharmaceutical industry) giving details of drugs and their side-effects. It is a useful guide, so long as it is not seen as the final word.
Monthly Index of Medical Specialities (MIMS). This is a monthly index of drugs that is handy for a quick reference to a drug name. There is very limited information about side-effects (*www.mims.com.au* is available bi-monthly).
Physicians Desk Reference (Montvale, NJ, USA, 1998).
Drug Information for the Health Care Professional (USPDI, 2001). This is an annual publication of adverse effects by US Pharmacopeia.
Advice for the Patient: Drug Information in Lay Language (USPDI).
Tarascon Pocket Pharmacopoeia: 2002 by Steven M. Green (Tarascon, 2002).
Saunders Drug Handbook for Health Professions by Robert, Kizior, Barbara and Hodgson (WB Saunders, 2001).

Other sources of information

Beyond Prozac by Dr Terry Lynch (Marino, 2001).
Toxic Psychiatry by Dr Peter Breggin (Harper Collins, 1993).
Your Drug May Be Your Problem by Dr Peter Breggin and Dr David Cohen (Perseus, 1999).

Internet

www.bnf.org – British National Formulary; a useful source of reliable drug information.

www.emc.vhn.net – *electronic* Medicines Compendium (eMC); provides data sheets and Summaries of Product Characteristics (SPCs). This covers 2,500 medicines licensed in the UK. You must register (for free) to use it.

www.regsource.com – a huge resource for information about medications, including links to regulatory authorities, pharmacology and pharmaceutical databases, medical information and much more.

http://www-sci.lib.uci.edu/~martindale/Pharmacy.html#HUMAN – an interesting catalogue of online information regarding pharmacology, pharmacy and more.

www.abpi.org.uk – website of the Association of the British Pharmaceutical Industry (ABPI), with links to individual pharmaceutical companies.

www.admin.safescript.com/drugcgic.cgi/START – The World Standard Drug Database has a searchable drug information database. You have to be careful what you ask and how you ask it. For example, I entered liver enzymes and had a relatively short list of drugs that cause abnormal liver enzymes. However, on searching for liver function tests, a much more comprehensive list emerged.

www.drugs.com is an online drug information resource with a searchable database.

www.medlineplus.gov gives health information for the public, including access to databases such as Medline.

www.medscape.com/druginfo gives access to two drug databases, including drug–drug and drug–food interactions.

www.mims.com.au is available bi-monthly in Australia.

www.nursespdr.com/members/database/ndrhtml/druglist.html is a comprehensive drug listing with searchable database.

www.pharmacy.org/company.html links to pharmaceutical companies worldwide.

www.pharmweb.net

www.rxlist.com is a useful index of drug information.

www.safemedication.com is run by the American Society of Health-System Pharmacists and gives good basic information about drugs.

www.stjames.ie/ClinicalInformation/NationalMedicinesInformationCentre is based at St. James' Hospital, Dublin, Ireland, and gives access to information about prescribed drugs.

www.thedrugmonitor.com is a not-for-profit site giving information about drug treatment to practitioners and students of medicine, pharmacy and other allied health sciences.

www.usp.org is the website of the US Pharmacopeia. This offers information on prescribed drugs, including their annual book publication, *Drug Information for the HealthCare Professional.*

Drug regulatory authorities

Ireland
Irish Medicines Board, Earlsfort Centre, Earlsfort Terrace, Dublin 2, Ireland
(email: *foi@imb.ie*; website: *www.imb.ie*).

UK
Committee on Safety of Medicines (CSM),
which provides information and advice to the UK Licensing Authority
(website: *www.mca.gov.uk/aboutagency/regframework/csm/csmhome.htm*).
Medicines Control Agency, Market Towers, 1Nine Elms Lane, London SW8 5NQ, UK
(email: *info@mca.gsi.gov.uk*; website: *www.mca.gov.uk*).

USA
US Food and Drug Administration, 5600 Fishers Lane, Rockville, MD 20857-0001, USA
(website: *www.fda.gov*).

Australia
Therapeutic Goods Administration, PO Box 100, WODEN ACT 2606, Australia
(email: *tga-information-officer@health.gov.au*; website: *www.health.gov.au/tga*).

Canada
Health Canada, 12th floor, Jeanne Mance Building, Tunney's Pasture, Ottawa,
Ontario, K1A 0K9 (website: *www.hc-sc.gc.ca*).

New Zealand
Medsafe, New Zealand Medicines and Medical Devices Safety Authority, PO Box 5013,
Wellington, New Zealand (website: *www.medsafe.govt.nz/index.asp*).

South Africa
Medicines Control Council, Private Bag X828, Pretoria, South Africa. Government of
South Africa website: *www.gov.za*. Ministry of Health
(website: *http://196.36.153.56/doh/*).

THE INTERNET

In the past few years, there has been an explosion both in the number of people who have access to the Internet and the amount of information available there. A major consideration for anyone searching for information is the need for discrimination – what is helpful and what is not?

Many patients are specifically told by their doctors not to look for information on the Internet. Partly this arises from a belief that patients would be confused by a bewildering mass of detailed information. Another, less positive, motivation for this advice may be that doctors, on occasion, become apprehensive when patients seek access to information in order to make informed decisions about their own treatment.

The world of medicine is rapidly changing. People are generally more questioning of their health-care practitioners. As more information becomes widely available, this can be of great benefit in the search for relief from illness and enhanced health. However, there is a need for clearly presented sources of information that are easily accessible and can be used by anyone to assess their own particular situation.

With this in mind, I have created an innovative website that provides information and support to health-care practitioners and to the general public. There are several aspects to the website that will be of interest to practitioners:

- Medical information based upon *The Clinical Medicine Guide – A Holistic Perspective*
- Information on prescribed drugs that supports this drug reference book
- Cases of people treated with Chinese medicine or with homoeopathy
- Supervision and support service for holistic practitioners
- Support for the Study Guide that accompanies *The Clinical Medicine Guide – A Holistic Perspective*
- Handy suggestion sheets on diet, relaxation, exercise, childbirth, etc.

Dr Stephen Gascoigne
The Clinic of Chinese Medicine
Glebe House, Ardfield, Clonakilty, Co. Cork, Ireland
Tel: +353 (0)23 40986 Fax: +353 (0)23 40985
Email: info@drgascoigne.com Website: www.drgascoigne.com

HOW TO RECOGNISE SERIOUS SYMPTOMS

It is essential that we know how to recognise a serious symptom so that we can practise safely and ensure that our patients receive the best of care. Although people are often worried that drug reduction may lead to serious consequences, this is unusual. You should particularly give attention to which category of drug you are dealing with as discussed in Chapter 3. The table below lists symptoms that would indicate a serious condition; that is, a situation where life may be threatened or there is a severe degree of limitation. If you understand the significance of a particular symptom, you can have confidence in your practice and decide when further support or referral is needed.

The seriousness of a symptom is dependent upon the degree of limitation of the person's activity or functioning. If health can be defined as freedom from limitation, then disease or a symptom is a limiting factor. A serious symptom, therefore, would be one that is severely limiting, life threatening or indicative of a worsening situation (i.e. progressive over a short period of time).

What do you do in a situation where a symptom may indicate a serious condition? The answer to this depends upon the degree of your experience and expertise. It is important to recognise your limitations as to what is and is not possible. You may be able to deal with such symptoms. On the other hand, you may need to refer the person to someone else. There may be a need for emergency hospitalisation. This is true in acute life-threatening conditions.

If the case is not so severe, there may be time to refer to someone who may be of help. This could be a conventional practitioner or possibly a holistic practitioner. Whatever the situation, it is essential to discuss the issues with the person who has come to see you for help. You may be able to help later for the underlying problems, whilst current circumstances require a different approach in the short term.

Symptom	Cause for concern
Anorexia	Severe, progressive, with mental symptoms of distorted body image
Anuria	Always
Appetite, increased	With weight loss, with mental symptoms of distorted body image
Belching	Not serious
Bleeding	Severe, persistent, recurrent, with pallor, sore throat and lymphatic gland enlargement
Bleeding, vaginal, inter-menstrual	Persistent, particularly around the menopause
Bleeding, vaginal, post-coital[59]	Persistent
Bleeding, vaginal, post-menopausal	Always (unless taking hormone replacement treatment)
Bleeding, vaginal, pre-pubertal	Always (consider sexual abuse)
Bleeding, vaginal, after childbirth	If heavy
Bloating, abdomen	Progressive
Body image disturbance	If associated with weight loss, amenorrhoea
Breathlessness	Severe, acute, progressive, with confusion, with cyanosis, pulse rate > 120 per minute, paroxysmal attacks occurring at night
Bruising	Severe, spontaneous
Bullae	Large
Constipation	Severe, progressive, with blood, alternates with diarrhoea
Convulsions	Always
Cough	Persistent, with blood, with breathlessness

Cyanosis	Always, unless in cold weather only involving, lips/extremities
Deafness	Short history, progressive
Dehydration	This may result from loss of fluids, e.g. diarrhoea and vomiting or lack of intake. In babies look for dry skin/lips, decreased skin elasticity, strong urine, scanty urine or even dry nappy, sleepy, lack of responsiveness. In older people there will be reported thirst also.
Delusions	Always
Diarrhoea	Severe, persistent, progressive, in the very young or old, with blood, with mucus, alternates with constipation
Dizziness	Severe, progressive
Ear, deformity	Severe
Ear, discharge	Long duration
Emotional symptoms, e.g. anxiety, fear, depression	If severe, with mental symptoms
Enuresis	Severe, especially if with incontinence in the day
Eye, discharge	Not if alone. Of concern if severe, prolonged and with pain in the eye
Eye, redness	Circumcorneal, with visual disturbance
Eye, soreness	Not if mild (of concern if pain rather than soreness especially with circumcorneal redness)
Facial weakness	With history of ear pain
Fainting	With exercise
Fever, mild	Perhaps 99 deg. F. – may indicate mild disease but could be the beginning of severe disease in a weak patient (i.e. vital energy too weak to generate fever)

Fever, prolonged	Most fevers last a day or so. If several days have elapsed, then this is of concern, as the patient is not strong enough to throw off the problem.
Fever, very high	103 deg. F and above. This indicates potentially severe disease. There is strong vital energy but the process may damage the patient.
Finger clubbing	Always
Flatulence	Not serious
Haematuria	Painless
Haemoptysis	Recurrent, older patient, smoker
Hallucinations	Always
Headache	Progressive, severe with short history, with other central nervous system symptoms
High blood pressure	If severe, especially if associated with oedema and proteinuria
Hoarseness	Persistent (more than three weeks)
Jaundice	Unless mild in newborn
Labour, delayed onset	If more than two weeks overdue (this is flexible because it is dependent upon the mother and the baby)
Labour, prolonged	If cervix not dilating, with exhaustion, with changes to foetal heart rate
Loss of consciousness	With exercise, not if short duration with specific trigger (see page 105)
Lumps, around or on the ear	Severe, if with redness, pain and deafness
Lumps, general	Short history, progressive
Lumps,, nodules in the skin	Short history, recent change, progressive, bleeding
Lymphatic gland enlargement	With pallor, bleeding and sore throat, progressive, moderately enlarged

Nausea	Severe
Numbness	Severe, progressive
Oedema	Acute, unilateral, severe, progressive, with cardiac symptoms, with renal symptoms
Pain	Severe
Pain, abdominal	Severe, with abdominal rigidity, with guarding, with rebound tenderness
Pain, chest	Severe, at rest, with vomiting, with rapid pulse and low blood pressure, long duration, increasing frequency of attacks, constant and dull
Pain, ear	Severe, with fever
Pain, eye	With visual disturbance
Pain, loin	Severe
Pain, urethra	Not serious
Pallor	Severe, with fainting, with marked light-headedness or dizziness
Palpitations	Pulse > 120 or < 50, with chest pain, oedema or loss of consciousness
Paralysis	Always
Periods, heavy	Persistent, frequent, with pallor and tiredness
Placental retention	If with heavy bleeding, if prolonged (over an hour)
Pregnancy, uterine pain	Always, unless at normal time for labour
Pregnancy, vaginal bleeding	Always
Proteinuria	With dysuria and backache, with high blood pressure

Pulse diagnosis (Chinese medicine) in acute fevers	If you treat a patient with an External Pathogenic Factor (EPF) and the pulse is superficial, floating and even overflowing, you would expect the pulse to moderate after treatment. If this does not occur it indicates that the EPF may be stronger than the upright Qi. Careful assessment of the case is then necessary, as treatment is likely to be difficult. The next thing to happen may be collapse of the person.
Skin, redness or weeping	Severe, large areas of skin surface
Sputum	Copious, green/yellow, blood-stained, frothy
Stiffness	Severe
Stridor	Always
Suicidal feelings	Always
Suicidal thoughts	Always
Symptom, severity	The stronger the symptoms (e.g. lots of diarrhoea, lots of vomiting) then the more likely they are to be potentially serious. However, be careful since weak patients have weak symptoms, e.g. pneumonia in the elderly or patients with AIDS may present only with breathlessness – no cough and no fever. It is important to assess each case carefully.
Symptoms, progression	Assess the direction of the pathology. By this I mean is it moving to internal organs or becoming more superficial? It is of concern if symptoms start to appear indicating pathology at a deeper level, e.g. in the case of the respiratory system this would be illustrated by sore throat with fever, cough, breathlessness and finally confusion – an effect on the deepest level (mental).
Symptoms, site	Are these in the superficial levels of the body or involving internal organs? If symptoms occur indicating pathology in the lung, kidney, liver, heart or central nervous system, then these are clearly more worrying. In terms of Chinese medicine, worry more if the symptoms are at deeper levels of the Taiyin, Shaoyin and Jueyin.

Tendency to catch colds	Not serious (but indicates a weakened immune system)
Thought disorders	If severe
Tingling	Severe, progressive
Tinnitus	Progressive
Tremor	Severe, progressive
Urgency	Severe, short history
Urination, dribbling	Severe, short history
Urination, frequent	Severe, short history
Vaginal discharge	Heavy, blood-stained
Veins, distended	In an abnormal site (e.g. neck when sitting, over the chest or abdominal wall)
Vertigo	Severe
Vesicles	Haemorrhagic
Vision, blurring	Progressive
Vision, double	Short history
Vision, spots or floaters	If localised area of blurring
Visual disturbance	Short history, progressive, with pain, with redness
Vomiting	Severe, persistent, progressive, in the very young or old, with blood, with food eaten days before, projectile, evidence of dehydration
Weight loss	Progressive, unexplained, with mental symptoms of distorted body image
Wheezing	If accompanied by breathlessness

Note

[1] Do not forget that it takes two to indulge in sexual intercourse. I know of a woman who had several invasive investigations for post-coital bleeding only to discover later that her partner had blood-streaked semen.

LIAISON WITH OTHER PRACTITIONERS

Liaison with other practitioners is an essential part of medical practice. There are several reasons for asking another professional about the person you are treating. You may wish to refer the person you have seen because you cannot treat the particular presenting problem. It may be because several treatment options are necessary and working with other practitioners is part of an overall management plan for that person. Perhaps you would like a degree of supervision from the other practitioner. Whatever the reason, it is helpful to know how to go about the practical matter of liaison.

It is much more helpful if you know the practitioner. A resource list is invaluable where you know people in your locality such as a homoeopath, osteopath, acupuncturist, herbalist, counsellor and so on. If you have had contact with them previously, any dealings now will be smoother.

The standard way of liaising professionally is by means of referral letter. This may not be necessary if you know the practitioner concerned and the case is not too involved. It is preferable to communicate by letter, at least initially, for other situations and particularly when dealing with conventional practitioners who you do not know. It is often helpful to have written records of such communications for inclusion in the case notes.

Below is a sample letter that may be of guidance. Always type such a letter on professional notepaper. The main points to bring out are:

- state the main issue to be dealt with
- say what you are intending to do about it
- describe what help or assistance you require
- offer to discuss the case further
- enclose literature about your therapy if necessary

The Clinic of Chinese Medicine
Ardfield
Clonakilty
Co. Cork
Ireland

Tel No.

Date

Dear

Re: Mr A.N.Other, 14 Any Street, Anywhere

This man came to see me recently for help with his symptoms of anxiety and depression. As you know, he was diagnosed with a minor depressive illness some years ago. His main difficulties at the moment are disturbed sleep, palpitations, sweating together with feelings of apprehension, anxiety and nervousness. When his symptoms are particularly strong he finds his work difficult to cope with. This is the type of condition that can respond to acupuncture and Chinese herbal medicine and I have arranged to see him for a course of treatment.

I would envisage that his improvement will be slow and that he would require help from other sources including counselling. I have given him a list of people who would be able to help.

He also wishes help in reducing his medication, which currently consists of:

Anafranil 25 mg three times daily
Nitrazepam one at night
Diazepam 5 mg three times daily

I would appreciate your help later when it is appropriate to deal with these. In the meantime I shall keep in touch about his progress.

If you would like to discuss this case, I can be contacted at the above address. I also enclose a leaflet giving information about acupuncture and Chinese herbal medicine.

Yours sincerely

Stephen Gascoigne

E